Somatic Exercises For Beginners

Embark on a transformative 28-day journey to manage stress, alleviate pain, and cultivate inner peace through gentle movement and mindfulness

Helen Talbott

Copyright © 2024 Helen Talbott

All rights reserved. No part of this book may be reproduced, stored in a retrieval system, or transmitted in any form or by any means, electronic, mechanical, photocopying, recording, or otherwise, without written permission from the author, except for the use of brief quotations in a book review.

Disclaimer

The information contained in this book is for educational purposes only and is not intended as a substitute for professional medical advice, diagnosis, or treatment. Always consult with your healthcare provider before beginning any new exercise program, especially if you have any existing medical conditions. The author and publisher disclaim any responsibility for any adverse effects or injuries arising from the use or misuse of the information contained within.

Reader discretion is advised. Some of the exercises described in this book may require physical exertion and could potentially cause discomfort or injury if performed incorrectly. Please listen to your body, modify exercises as needed, and stop immediately if you experience any pain or discomfort.

"Start small, like a tiny seed growing into a mighty tree. Every mindful movement nourishes your connection to your body and strengthens your well-being."

Table of contents

I. Introduction:

- What are Somatic Exercises?
- Benefits of Somatic Exercises
- Who can benefit from this book?

II. Cultivating Harmony between Body and Mind:

- The mind-body connection and its impact on overall well-being
- Understanding the role of the nervous system in stress and trauma
- How somatic exercises can bridge the gap between mind and body

III. Fundamental and Scientific Principles of Somatic Exercises:

- Key principles of somatic movement: awareness, breathwork, gentle exploration
- The science behind the benefits: studies on stress reduction, pain management, and trauma recovery

- Different types of somatic practices

IV. Addressing Trauma Through Somatic Practices:

- Understanding the impact of trauma on the body and mind
- How somatic exercises can support the healing process
- Specific exercises for trauma recovery

V. Overcoming Common Challenges:

- Addressing common concerns about starting somatic exercises
- Tips for creating a safe and supportive practice environment
- Importance of self-compassion and building trust in your body

VI. Establishing a Secure Environment: Preparing for Somatic Exercises:

- Choosing the right environment and clothing

- Setting realistic expectations and intentions
- Warming up and preparing the body for movement

VII. Exercises for Stress and Anxiety Reduction:

- Gentle body scans for relaxation and awareness
- Breathwork exercises to calm the nervous system
- Movement sequences to release tension and promote grounding

VIII. Exercises for Trauma Recovery:

- Trauma-informed movement practices to promote safety and comfort
- Guided visualizations for emotional release and self-compassion
- Somatic meditations for processing and integrating experiences

IX. Exercises for Enhancing Flexibility and Relieving Tension:

- Gentle stretches and mobilizations for improved range of motion
- Exercises to release tension in specific areas
- Self-massage techniques for promoting relaxation and circulation

X. Alleviating Pain Through Somatic Exercises:

- Understanding the mind-body connection in chronic pain
- How somatic exercises can help manage pain
- Specific exercises for different types of pain

XI. Exercises for Improving Posture:

- Understanding the importance of good posture for stress reduction and pain management
- Exercises to strengthen core muscles and improve alignment
- Techniques for mindful movement and posture awareness

XII. Your 28-Day Somatic Program:

- A week-by-week breakdown of exercises for different goals
- Tips for integrating somatic practices into daily life
- Bonus

About the author page

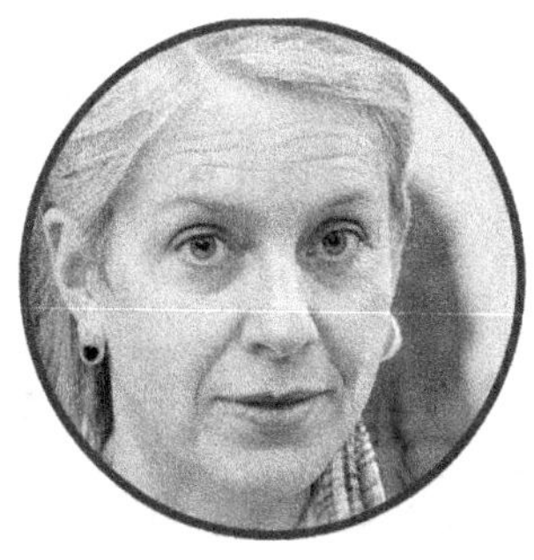

Helen Talbott isn't just an author; she's a guide, a passionate advocate for embodied living. Her journey began with a yearning for deeper understanding of her own body and its connection to her mind and emotions. Frustrated by traditional fitness routines that felt rigid and impersonal, she discovered the transformative power of somatic exercises. This exploration sparked a lifelong commitment to learning, sharing, and empowering others to reconnect with their bodies and unlock their innate potential for healing and well-being.

As Helen delves deeper into the world of somatic practices, she finds herself constantly learning from various disciplines, including dance, yoga, mindfulness, and bodywork therapies. This diverse background fuels her unique perspective and informs her approach to teaching and writing. Her writing style is characterized by gentle warmth, clear explanations, and a touch of humor, making even complex concepts accessible and engaging for beginners.

Beyond the written word, Helen actively shares her passion through workshops, retreats, and online communities. Witnessing the positive transformations experienced by her students is a constant source of inspiration and reinforces her belief in the power of somatic practices to empower individuals and foster a more connected, compassionate world.

When not guiding others on their somatic journeys, Helen can be found exploring the world through mindful movement, enjoying the quiet moments of nature, or simply savoring a cup of tea with a good book.

"Our bodies hold a wealth of wisdom, waiting to be unlocked. Through somatic exploration, we can learn to listen to this wisdom, move with intention, and cultivate a deeper sense of connection to ourselves and the world around us."

The mirror reflected a stranger - someone I didn't recognize. My body, once a canvas for carefree adventures, now felt like a prison, weighed down by stress and neglect. Every movement was a chore, a reminder of the disconnect between my mind and flesh. I knew I needed a change, but the gym felt intimidating, the diets restrictive, and the fads unsustainable. Then, I stumbled upon something different: somatic movement.

It wasn't about sculpted abs or calorie counting. It was about listening, feeling, and reconnecting with my body as a whole. The first class was awkward. We moved slowly, focusing on the sensations in our feet as we walked, the breath in our lungs, the way our muscles engaged with the ground. It felt strange, almost childlike, but a spark ignited within me.

As weeks turned into months, the awkwardness melted away. I began to discover a language within my body, a vocabulary of sensations I never knew existed. The tightness in my shoulders released with gentle stretches, the knot in my stomach softened with mindful breathing. I wasn't just moving; I was having a conversation, a dialogue between my inner world and the physical form it inhabited.

The changes weren't just physical. My mind, once clouded with anxiety, began to find stillness. The constant chatter quieted, replaced by a sense of quiet awareness. I carried this newfound peace throughout my day, responding to stress with calm instead of reactivity. My relationships deepened as I learned to listen not just with my ears, but with my whole being.

My somatic journey wasn't easy. There were days when old patterns crept in, days when the disconnect felt overwhelming. But with each practice, I learned to be patient, to acknowledge the pain and move through it. I found support in a community of like-minded individuals, each on their own path of rediscovery.

Today, the stranger in the mirror is fading. I see myself, not as a perfect image, but as a work in progress, a being constantly evolving and learning. My body is no longer a prison, but a vessel for exploration and joy. And the journey continues, each movement a brushstroke on the canvas of my life, a testament to the power of listening, feeling, and becoming whole.

My descent into disconnection had been gradual, like a slow leak in a tire. The constant hum of stress, the ache in my shoulders, the chronic fatigue – I'd become numb to it all. Exercise felt like another chore, another box to tick on a list that never seemed to get shorter. My body, once a source of boundless energy and exploration, had become a stranger, a vessel I navigated on autopilot.

Then, a friend mentioned somatic movement. The name itself held a certain mystique, an invitation to something deeper than sculpted abs or calorie counting. Intrigued, I delved deeper. I learned about the focus on internal sensations, the exploration of movement as a dialogue with your body, not just a means to an end. A spark flickered within me, a yearning for something I couldn't quite articulate.

But it wasn't just the theoretical underpinnings that drew me in. It was the stories. People talked about finding relief from chronic pain, unearthing emotions they'd buried deep, rediscovering a sense of joy in movement. They spoke of a reconnection, a homecoming to their own bodies, and that resonated with a desperate ache within me.

The first class was a revelation. Gone were the mirrors, the pounding music, the pressure to perform. Instead, there was quietness, introspection, and a gentle invitation to listen. We moved slowly, focusing on the subtle shifts in our weight as we walked, the way our breath danced in our lungs, the almost imperceptible tremor in our muscles. It felt strange, almost ridiculously simple, yet a profound curiosity bloomed within me.

As the weeks unfolded, the awkwardness dissolved. I began to discover a language within my body, a vocabulary of sensations I never knew existed. The tightness in my chest softened with mindful breathing, the tension in my jaw released with gentle stretches. Each movement wasn't just an exercise; it was a conversation, a peeling back of layers to reveal the being beneath the stress and strain.

The impact wasn't confined to the physical. My mind, once a churning vortex of anxieties, started to find moments of stillness. The constant chatter quieted, replaced by a deep sense of presence. I carried this newfound peace into my daily life, responding to challenges with calm instead of reactivity. My relationships deepened as I learned to listen not just with my ears, but with my whole being.

Somatic movement wasn't a quick fix, a magic bullet for all my problems. There were days when old patterns resurfaced, days when the disconnect felt overwhelming. But with each practice, I learned to be patient, to acknowledge the pain and move through it. I found support in a community of like-minded individuals, each on their own path of rediscovery.

Today, I'm still on that journey, each movement a brushstroke on the canvas of my life. The stranger in the mirror is fading, replaced by a deeper sense of self, a being constantly evolving and learning. Somatic movement wasn't just a new exercise routine; it was an invitation, a doorway to a deeper understanding of myself, my body, and the world around me. And the journey continues, fueled by the spark of curiosity that ignited all those months ago.

My foray into somatic movement wasn't a walk in the park – not by a long shot. Sure, the idea of gentle exploration and reconnecting with my body sounded idyllic, but the reality was far more nuanced, filled with unexpected hurdles and moments of self-doubt.

One of the biggest challenges was **breaking free from old habits**. Decades of pushing my body through rigid workouts, ignoring its whispers of discomfort, had left deep grooves in my physical and mental landscape. It was hard to let go of the "no pain, no gain" mentality and embrace the slower, gentler pace of somatic movement. Sometimes, the urge to crank up the intensity or push myself to the limit would come knocking, and I had to gently remind myself that this was a different journey, one built on listening and respecting my body's wisdom.

Then there was the **emotional rollercoaster**. As I started tuning into my body's sensations, long-buried emotions began to surface. Memories I had tucked away, anxieties I had suppressed, all came flooding back, sometimes triggered by a simple movement or breathwork exercise. It was uncomfortable, raw, and often left me feeling overwhelmed. But with the support of my instructor and the understanding community I found, I learned to navigate these emotional waves, allowing them to flow through me without judgment.

Another hurdle was the **constant comparison trap**. Social media, with its filtered images of perfectly toned bodies and seemingly effortless movement, played its insidious role. Seeing others seemingly "master" somatic practices while I still fumbled with the basics triggered feelings of inadequacy and self-doubt. It took a conscious effort to shift my focus inwards, to celebrate my own unique journey and progress, and to remember that everyone's path is different.

Despite the challenges, there were moments of pure magic. The first time I felt a knot of tension in my shoulders release with a simple breath, the first time I moved with a newfound sense of ease and fluidity – these experiences were transformative. They fueled my motivation, reminding me of the power and potential of somatic movement to heal and reconnect.

Looking back, I realize that the challenges were an integral part of the journey. They forced me to go deeper, to confront my limitations and push past them. They taught me valuable lessons about self-compassion, patience, and the importance of listening to my body's unique needs. And ultimately, they made the transformation all the more meaningful.

The beauty of somatic movement lies in its diverse practices, each offering unique pathways to explore your inner landscape. For me, several specific exercises left a lasting impact, each resonating with different aspects of my journey:

1. Breathwork: This wasn't just about taking deep breaths. We practiced various techniques, focusing on the rise and fall of the abdomen, the subtle expansion and contraction of the ribcage, and the way the breath danced in our nostrils. This simple act of observing my breath became a powerful tool for grounding myself, calming anxieties, and accessing a deeper sense of presence.

2. Floor rolling: Imagine gently rolling around on the floor like a child, exploring the sensations on your skin, the way your muscles engage and release. This playful practice, often accompanied by guided imagery, helped me release tension I didn't even know I held, fostering a sense of lightness and ease in my body.

3. Guided movement explorations: These weren't your typical workout routines. We explored simple movements like walking, reaching, bending, focusing on the internal sensations, the subtle shifts in weight distribution, the articulation of each joint. It was like rediscovering the joy of movement, free from judgment and striving, simply for the sake of experiencing.

4. Partner exercises: Working with a partner, we engaged in gentle mirroring exercises, responding to their movements without judgment. This practice fostered a deep sense of connection, both with myself and with another human being, reminding me of the inherent social nature of movement.

5. Mindfulness meditation: While not strictly a "movement" practice, incorporating mindfulness meditations into my routine helped me cultivate a deeper awareness of my body, my emotions, and my thoughts. This awareness became a cornerstone of my somatic journey, allowing me to navigate challenges with greater clarity and compassion.

These are just a few examples, and what resonates most with you will be unique to your own journey. The key is to explore, experiment, and be open to the unexpected ways these practices can unlock transformation within you. Remember, the most profound impact often lies in the seemingly simple things, the gentle invitations to listen, feel, and reconnect with the wisdom of your own body.

My somatic journey wasn't just about stretching and breathing exercises; it was a ripple effect that touched every aspect of my life. It started with the physical, of course. My chronic pain lessened, my posture improved, and I moved with a newfound ease I hadn't known I missed. But the impact went far beyond that.

The mental shift: The constant chatter in my head, the anxiety that used to gnaw at me, started to fade. With each mindful breath, each gentle movement exploration, I learned to quiet the noise and find a sense of inner peace. This newfound calmness spilled over into my daily life, allowing me to approach challenges with more clarity and less reactivity.

Relationships deepened: My somatic journey taught me the power of truly listening, not just with my ears, but with my whole being. This newfound awareness translated into my relationships, both personal and professional. I became more attuned to the needs of others, more present in conversations, and more able to build genuine connections.

Creative spark ignited: As I reconnected with my body, a long-dormant creativity reawakened. I found myself drawn to writing, painting, and other forms of artistic expression. The somatic practices, with their emphasis on inner exploration and sensory awareness, opened up new pathways for creativity to flow.

Confidence blossomed: As I shed the layers of self-doubt and learned to appreciate my body for what it was, not what it should be, my confidence blossomed. I started saying "no" more often, setting boundaries, and prioritizing my well-being. This newfound self-respect permeated all areas of my life, from my career to my relationships.

Gratitude overflowed: The more I tuned into my body, the more I began to appreciate its incredible capabilities. Each breath, each heartbeat, became a testament to the miracle of life. This deep sense of gratitude infused my every interaction, filling my life with a newfound joy and appreciation.

My somatic journey wasn't a quick fix or a magical solution to all my problems. It was, and continues to be, a process of exploration, self-discovery, and learning. But the impact it's had on my life is undeniable. It's opened up a world of possibilities, reminding me that the journey of self-discovery is never-ending, and the body holds the key to unlocking our full potential. And as I continue on this path, I do so with a heart full of gratitude for the transformation it has brought and the exciting possibilities that lie ahead.

Chapter 1

Introduction

Imagine Waking up with a smile, your body humming with ease, and a sense of calm washing over you even in the face of daily chaos.

This isn't some distant dream, but a reality waiting to be unlocked through the power of **somatic exercises**. Forget the grueling gym routines and forced push-ups. This journey is about **listening**, **feeling**, and **gently guiding your body** towards a state of **mind-body harmony**.

Tired of stress and anxiety gripping your days? Somatic exercises can melt that tension away, leaving you feeling grounded and present. **Do chronic aches and pains cast a shadow over your life?** These gentle movements can help you reclaim your body, releasing stored trauma and restoring its natural ease. **Yearning**

for a deeper connection to yourself? Somatic practices offer a unique path to self-discovery, where your body becomes a map to your inner wisdom.

This book is your **28-day passport** to this transformative journey. Whether you're a complete beginner or just curious about a different approach to movement, we'll guide you every step of the way. You'll learn about the science behind somatic exercises, discover how they can address trauma, and practice gentle yet powerful exercises tailored to your specific needs. We'll create a safe space for exploration, equip you with tools for self-compassion, and celebrate your progress as you rediscover the joy of movement and the profound connection between your body and mind.

Are you ready to embark on a journey towards a calmer, stronger, and more connected you? Turn the page and let's begin.

What are Somatic Exercises: Unraveling the Mind-Body Connection

Imagine movement that's not a chore, but a conversation; not about pushing harder, but about **listening deeper**. Enter the world of **somatic exercises**, a practice as gentle as a butterfly landing and as powerful as a wave washing over the shore. But what exactly are they?

Somatic exercises are more than just stretches and bends. They're a unique approach to movement that **bridges the gap between your mind and body**. Unlike traditional fitness routines focused on achieving external goals, somatic practices turn inwards, emphasizing **awareness, sensation, and gentle exploration.**

Think of it this way: Your body holds stories, both joyful and painful. Stressful experiences leave their mark in clenched muscles and shallow breaths. Through somatic exercises, you become a detective, carefully observing these sensations without judgment. By **tuning into the subtleties of your body**, you begin to unravel these stories, releasing tension and rediscovering your natural ease of movement.

Here are some key aspects of somatic exercises:

1. Cultivating Awareness: It all starts with noticing. Somatic exercises guide you to pay attention to subtle sensations in your body – the way your feet feel on the ground, the stretch in your muscles, the rhythm of your breath. This heightened awareness becomes your compass, guiding your movements and revealing areas of tension.

2. Gentle Exploration: Forget forced stretches and gym routines. Somatic exercises are **slow, gentle, and explorative**. Instead of pushing towards an idealized end result, you focus on the present moment, experimenting with small movements and observing their impact. This gentle approach allows your body to release tension and rediscover its natural movement patterns.

3. Mind-Body Integration: Somatic exercises recognize that your mind and body are not separate entities, but a beautifully intertwined system. As you explore movement with awareness, you also become aware of your thoughts and emotions. This integration allows you to address negative thought patterns and emotional blocks that hold tension in your body, leading to more holistic well-being.

4. Embodied Trauma Release: Trauma can leave its mark not just emotionally, but also physically, manifesting as chronic pain, tension, and restricted movement. Somatic exercises offer a safe and gentle way to release this stored trauma. By bringing awareness to these areas, you can gradually work through them, promoting healing and reclaiming your body's natural ease.

5. A Journey, not a Destination: Somatic exercises are not about achieving perfection or reaching a specific goal. It's a journey of exploration, self-discovery, and developing a deeper relationship with your body. Be patient, be kind to yourself, and celebrate the small victories along the way.

Exploring Different Somatic Practices:

Somatic exercises encompass a wide range of practices, each with its own unique approach. Some popular methods include:

- **Feldenkrais:** Uses gentle movements and guided awareness to improve mobility and ease chronic pain.
- **Alexander Technique:** Focuses on improving posture and movement awareness in everyday activities.
- **Laban Movement Analysis:** Explores the expressive qualities of movement and their connection to emotions.
- **Body-Mind Centering:** Connects with the deeper structures of the body through gentle movement and visualization.

Ready to Embark on your Somatic Journey?

Somatic exercises offer a powerful gateway to a calmer, more connected you. Remember, **you don't need to be a yogi or have any special skills to begin**. All you need is an open mind, a willingness to listen to your body, and a desire to move differently. With this book as your guide, you'll have the tools and knowledge to embark on this transformative journey. So, take a deep breath, step onto the mat, and begin your exploration of the incredible world of somatic exercises. The journey starts now.

Unveiling the Jewel Box: Benefits of Somatic Exercises

Imagine a toolbox overflowing with treasures, each offering a key to unlock a healthier, happier you. That's the essence of **somatic exercises**, a practice that goes beyond physical movement and delves into the enriching realm of **mind-body connection**. But what gems does this toolbox hold? Let's explore the diverse benefits of somatic exercises:

1. **Stress & Anxiety Relief:** Feeling overwhelmed by the daily grind? Somatic exercises can be your stress-busting allies. By tuning into your body's sensations, you learn to **identify and release tension** held in muscles and tissues. Gentle movements and breathwork activate the relaxation response, calming your nervous system and washing away anxiety. Studies show significant reductions in stress hormones like cortisol, promoting inner peace and emotional stability.

2. Pain Management & Healing: Chronic pain can be a debilitating shadow, but somatic exercises offer a ray of hope. By bringing awareness to pain areas, you gain insights into their causes and learn to release the physical tension associated with them. Gentle movements and self-massage techniques can improve circulation and flexibility, easing pain and promoting healing. This approach is particularly beneficial for conditions like back pain, headaches, and fibromyalgia.

3. Trauma Recovery & Emotional Integration: Traumas leave their mark not just emotionally, but also physically. Somatic exercises offer a safe and gentle way to **release stored trauma** held in the body. By observing sensations without judgment, you can begin to process and release emotional blocks, promoting healing and reclaiming your sense of safety and well-being. This approach is powerful for individuals dealing with PTSD, anxiety, and emotional distress.

4. Enhanced Flexibility & Mobility: Stiff and creaky joints? Somatic exercises can unlock your body's natural ease of movement. Unlike stretching routines that push beyond your limits, these practices emphasize gentle exploration and awareness. As you move mindfully, you'll discover areas of restriction and gradually increase your range of motion, leading to improved flexibility and agility.

5. Deeper Self-Awareness & Connection: Somatic exercises invite you to become an observer of your own body, a detective uncovering its hidden stories. By paying attention to your sensations, thoughts, and emotions, you develop a deeper understanding of yourself. This self-awareness empowers you to make conscious choices, manage stress effectively, and cultivate a stronger sense of self-compassion.

6. Improved Posture & Body Mechanics: Poor posture can lead to aches, pains, and a diminished sense of confidence. Somatic exercises teach you to move with awareness, aligning your body in a natural and balanced way. You'll learn to engage the right muscles for everyday activities, reducing strain and improving your overall posture.

7. Enhanced Creativity & Expressive Movement: Somatic exercises go beyond just physical benefits. By exploring movement with awareness, you tap into the expressive potential of your body. This can lead to increased creativity, improved coordination, and a deeper connection to your artistic side.

8. Stress-Free Exercise: Forget the pressure of gym routines and calorie counting. Somatic exercises are gentle and non-competitive, suitable for people of all ages and fitness levels. They offer a stress-free way to move your body and nourish your well-being, leaving you feeling energized and refreshed.

9. Cultivating Gratitude & Mindfulness: As you practice somatic exercises, you develop a keen appreciation for your body's incredible capabilities. This deepens your sense of gratitude and cultivates a mindful approach to everyday movement. You become more present in the moment, savoring the experience of being alive.

10. A Life-Long Journey of Discovery: Somatic exercises are not a quick fix, but a lifelong journey of self-discovery and growth. By incorporating these practices into your daily life, you continuously learn about yourself, unlock new possibilities for movement, and cultivate a deeper connection to your mind and body.

Remember, the benefits of somatic exercises are not confined to this list. As you embark on this transformative journey, you may discover unexpected treasures within yourself, unlocking a path towards a healthier, happier, and more authentic you. So, open the toolbox of somatic exercises, explore its diverse offerings, and unlock the gems waiting to enrich your life!

Who Can Benefit from This Book: Unlocking Your Somatic Potential

Do you ever find yourself longing for a calmer, more connected you? Do you yearn to move with ease, manage stress more effectively, and unlock the wisdom held within your body? If you answered yes, then this book on somatic exercises is for **you**.

Here's why:

1. The Stressed and Overwhelmed: If daily pressures leave you feeling anxious, exhausted, and disconnected from your body, somatic exercises offer a powerful antidote. By learning to listen to your body's subtle cues and release tension through gentle movement, you can cultivate inner peace and navigate stress with greater ease.

2. The Pain Warriors: Whether you struggle with chronic pain, headaches, or post-injury stiffness, somatic exercises can be your ally. By exploring movement with awareness and releasing held tension, you can gain insights into your pain's root cause and find gentle ways to manage and reduce it.

3. The Trauma Survivors: The impact of trauma often lingers in the body long after the emotional wounds have healed. Somatic exercises offer a safe and compassionate space to explore these stored tensions, process emotional blocks, and gradually reclaim a sense of safety and well-being in your body.

4. The Movement Seekers: Whether you're a fitness enthusiast or simply enjoy moving your body, somatic exercises can offer a fresh perspective. By emphasizing mindful exploration and gentle movement, you can discover new ways to move with ease, improve your flexibility, and unlock the expressive potential of your body.

5. The Curious Explorers: Are you fascinated by the mind-body connection and eager to learn more about yourself? Somatic exercises offer a unique journey of self-discovery. As you explore your body's sensations and movement patterns, you gain a deeper understanding of your thoughts, emotions, and overall well-being.

6. The Everyday Heroes: This book is not just for those with specific challenges. The principles of somatic exercises can benefit **everyone**. Whether you're a busy professional, a stay-at-home parent, or an athlete, incorporating these practices into your daily life can enhance your well-being, improve your posture, and cultivate a deeper sense of connection to yourself.

Remember, you don't need to be a yogi or an athlete to benefit from this book. All you need is an open mind, a willingness to listen to your body, and a desire to move differently. This book will be your guide, offering clear instructions, accessible exercises, and valuable insights on the transformative power of somatic practices.

So, are you ready to unlock your somatic potential? Turn the page and embark on a

journey towards a calmer, more connected, and more authentic you!

The Mind-Body Symphony: Unveiling the Interconnectedness of Our Being

For centuries, we've been taught to think of our minds and bodies as separate entities. However, modern science and ancient wisdom converge on a powerful truth: our minds and bodies are not isolated islands, but rather **intertwined elements composing a single, magnificent symphony**. This intricate connection, known as the **mind-body connection**, significantly impacts our overall well-being, influencing our physical health, emotional state, and overall sense of harmony.

Imagine your mind as the conductor, orchestrating the movements of your body, directing your thoughts, and shaping your emotions. Your body, in turn, acts as the orchestra, responding to the conductor's cues with physical sensations, physiological changes, and emotional responses. This interplay is constant, dynamic, and profoundly impactful.

How does the mind-body connection affect our well-being?

1. Stress and Anxiety: Chronic stress throws the symphony into disarray. Negative thoughts and anxieties trigger the release of stress hormones, causing physiological changes like increased heart rate, muscle tension, and shallow breathing. These physical responses further fuel anxiety, creating a vicious cycle that can negatively impact sleep, digestion, and overall health.

2. Pain and Chronic Conditions: Studies have shown that chronic pain can be amplified by negative thoughts and emotions. Conversely, mindfulness practices and positive thinking can reduce pain perception. This highlights the mind's ability to influence physical sensations, suggesting the potential of mind-body therapies for managing pain.

3. Emotional Well-being: Our physical health impacts our emotions. Poor sleep can lead to irritability, while chronic pain can contribute to depression. Conversely, physical activity and healthy eating can boost mood and emotional resilience. This demonstrates how nurturing our bodies can positively impact our emotional well-being.

4. Overall Sense of Harmony: When our minds and bodies are in sync, we experience a sense of wholeness and well-being. Our thoughts are clear, our bodies are relaxed, and our emotions are balanced. This harmony allows us to navigate challenges with greater resilience, enjoy life more fully, and live with a sense of purpose.

Exploring the Symphony: How to Cultivate the Mind-Body Connection:

Thankfully, the mind-body connection is not a passive force. We can actively cultivate it through various practices:

- **Mindfulness:** By focusing on the present moment, observing our thoughts and sensations without judgment, we gain awareness of the mind-body connection and learn to regulate our responses.

- **Physical Activity:** Exercise releases endorphins, natural mood enhancers, and improves blood flow, promoting physical and emotional well-being.
- **Yoga and Meditation:** These practices combine physical postures, breathing techniques, and mindfulness, fostering relaxation, stress reduction, and self-awareness.
- **Creative Expression:** Engaging in art, music, or dance allows us to connect with our emotions, express ourselves authentically, and promote emotional well-being.
- **Healthy Habits:** Eating nutritious foods, getting enough sleep, and spending time in nature nourish both body and mind, creating a foundation for overall well-being.

By incorporating these practices into your life, you become the conductor of your own symphony. You learn to listen to your body's whispers, guide your thoughts with intention, and cultivate a harmonious interplay between your mind and body. Remember, this journey is not about achieving perfection, but about fostering a mindful, compassionate relationship with yourself, allowing the symphony of your being to play its most beautiful melody.

Embrace the interconnectedness of your mind and body, and witness the transformative power it holds for your overall well-being. Start tuning your symphony today, and experience the joy of a life lived in harmony.

Chapter 2

Cultivating Harmony between Body and Mind

The Nervous System: Conductor of Stress and Trauma's Orchestra

Imagine a complex orchestra, with instruments representing the many parts of your body. The conductor, wielding immense power, is your **nervous system**: the maestro orchestrating your response to every experience, be it a gentle breeze or a roaring lion. Understanding its role in stress and trauma is crucial for navigating these challenges and fostering well-being.

The Two Main Players:

- **Sympathetic Nervous System (SNS):** This is your "fight-or-flight" conductor. When faced with stress or danger, it kicks in, preparing your body for action: increased heart rate, faster breathing, and heightened alertness. This response is essential for survival, allowing you to react quickly to threats.

- **Parasympathetic Nervous System (PNS):** This is your "rest-and-digest" conductor. When the threat subsides, it takes over, calming your body down and promoting relaxation, digestion, and regeneration.

Stress & The Symphony's Discord:

Chronic stress throws the orchestra into disarray. The SNS becomes overactive, constantly preparing for a perceived threat, even if one doesn't exist. This leads to:

- **Muscle tension:** The orchestra's instruments remain tightly strung, leading to headaches, neck pain, and other physical symptoms.
- **Digestive issues:** The focus shifts from digestion to fight-or-flight, causing problems like constipation or irritable bowel syndrome.

- **Sleep disturbances:** The calming PNS struggles to take over, leading to insomnia and fatigue.
- **Emotional dysregulation:** The conductor loses control, leading to anxiety, irritability, and difficulty managing emotions.

Trauma & The Symphony's Scars:

Trauma can leave lasting imprints on the nervous system, like scars on the orchestra's instruments. The SNS might become overly sensitive, triggering a fight-or-flight response even to harmless triggers. The PNS might struggle to function, leaving the body in a constant state of tension and hypervigilance. This can lead to:

- **Chronic pain:** The orchestra remains tense, leading to widespread pain and discomfort.
- **Flashbacks and nightmares:** The trauma replaying in the mind disrupts the

orchestra, causing intrusive memories and sleep disturbances.

- **Hypervigilance and anxiety:** The conductor remains on edge, scanning for potential threats, leading to constant worry and fear.
- **Emotional dysregulation:** The orchestra's instruments are out of tune, leading to difficulty managing emotions and expressing feelings.

Healing the Symphony: Regaining Harmony:

The good news is that the nervous system is not set in stone. By incorporating tools like:

- **Somatic exercises:** These gentle movements help release tension held in the body, allowing the orchestra to relax and recalibrate.
- **Mindfulness and meditation:** These practices calm the mind and promote awareness of the body's sensations, helping the conductor regain control.

- **Deep breathing:** Slow, diaphragmatic breathing activates the PNS, promoting relaxation and calming the orchestra's frantic pace.
- **Trauma-informed therapy:** This specialized therapy helps individuals process and integrate traumatic experiences, allowing the orchestra to heal from its scars.

By nurturing your nervous system and fostering mind-body connection, you can become the conductor of your own healing journey. With patience, practice, and the right tools, you can restore harmony to your symphony, leading to a life filled with greater peace, resilience, and well-being.

Remember: The nervous system is an intricate and powerful network. While this explanation offers a simplified overview, it's crucial to seek professional guidance if you are experiencing significant stress or trauma. With support and self-compassion, you can help your internal orchestra play its most beautiful melody yet.

Building the Bridge: How Somatic Exercises Connect Mind and Body

For centuries, we've been conditioned to think of mind and body as separate entities. However, the reality is far more interconnected, and **somatic exercises** offer a unique bridge to cultivate harmony between these seemingly distinct parts of our being.

Imagine your mind as a bustling city, with thoughts and emotions swirling like traffic. Your body is the vast landscape surrounding it, with sensations and physical experiences playing out like weather patterns. Somatic exercises act as bridges, allowing you to cross from the mental cityscape to the physical landscape, fostering a deeper understanding and connection.

Here's how somatic exercises bridge the mind-body gap:

1. Tuning into the Body's Whispers: Somatic exercises focus on **gentle movement and mindful awareness**. You learn to pay attention to subtle sensations in your body, like the way your feet connect to the ground, the tension in your muscles, or the rhythm of your breath. This heightened awareness acts as a bridge, allowing the mind to become attuned to the body's whispers, often ignored in the daily hustle.

2. Releasing Held Tension: Stress and trauma leave their mark not just emotionally, but also physically, manifesting as tension in muscles and tissues. Somatic exercises, through gentle movements and self-exploration, help you release this stored tension. As the physical tension melts away, it creates space for emotional release, fostering a deeper connection between mind and body.

3. Exploring the Landscape of Movement: Traditional exercise routines often focus on achieving external goals, disconnecting us from the internal experience. Somatic exercises, however, encourage **gentle exploration**. You experiment with small movements, observing their impact on your body and mind. This exploration becomes a bridge, allowing you to discover hidden aspects of yourself, both physically and emotionally.

4. Embodied Emotions: Emotions are not just mental experiences, but also have physical manifestations. Somatic exercises allow you to **connect emotions to physical sensations**. For example, noticing tightness in your chest might indicate anger, while feeling grounded in your feet could suggest a sense of security. This embodied awareness becomes a bridge, allowing you to process emotions on a deeper level, integrating them both physically and mentally.

5. Breaking the Habitual: We often get stuck in repetitive physical and mental patterns. Somatic exercises invite you to **step outside these patterns**. By experimenting with new movements and observing your reactions, you break free from automatic responses. This mindful exploration becomes a bridge, allowing you to create new connections between mind and body, fostering greater flexibility and adaptability.

The Journey Across the Bridge:

The bridge built by somatic exercises is not a destination, but a lifelong journey. As you continue to explore, you'll discover:

- **Improved stress management:** By releasing tension and cultivating awareness, you gain tools to manage stress and navigate daily challenges with greater ease.
- **Enhanced self-awareness:** As you connect with your body's sensations and emotions, you develop a deeper understanding of yourself, your needs, and your values.
- **Greater resilience:** By fostering mind-body harmony, you become more resilient to life's inevitable challenges, allowing you to bounce back from setbacks with greater ease.
- **A sense of wholeness:** When mind and body are in sync, you experience a profound sense of wholeness and

well-being, allowing you to live a more authentic and fulfilling life.

So, take a deep breath, step onto the bridge, and embark on your own journey of somatic exploration. As you connect with your body's wisdom and explore the landscape of your being, you'll witness the transformative power of bridging the gap between mind and body, leading you towards a life filled with greater harmony, self-compassion, and well-being.

chapter 3

Fundamental and Scientific Principles of Somatic Exercises

Unveiling the Key Principles of Somatic Movement: A Journey Within

Somatic movement isn't just about stretching and strengthening; it's a profound exploration of the mind-body connection. Unlike traditional fitness routines, it focuses on gentle awareness, listening, and exploration, unlocking a deeper understanding of ourselves and our movement patterns. Let's delve into the key principles that guide this transformative practice:

1. **Awareness:** At the heart of somatic movement lies **mindful awareness**. You learn to tune into subtle sensations in your body, like the way your breath moves through your lungs, the contact of your feet with the ground, or the subtle shifts in muscle tension. This heightened

awareness becomes a gateway, allowing you to connect with yourself on a deeper level and observe how your body responds to movement.

2. Gentle Exploration: Forget pushing your limits or achieving external goals. Somatic movement emphasizes **gentle and curious exploration**. You experiment with small, mindful movements, observing their impact on your body and mind. This exploration is non-judgmental, allowing you to discover hidden aspects of yourself, both physically and emotionally.

3. Embodied Learning: Traditional exercise often separates mind and body. Somatic practices, however, encourage **embodied learning**. You experience movement not just physically, but also emotionally and cognitively. This holistic approach allows you to integrate new information and skills on a deeper level, leading to lasting change.

4. Respectful Inquiry: Somatic movement fosters an attitude of **respectful inquiry**. You approach your body with curiosity and kindness, avoiding judgment or forcing yourself into uncomfortable positions. This respectful approach creates a safe space for exploration and allows you to discover your body's natural limits and capacities.

5. Integration & Release: Somatic movement recognizes that our bodies hold onto past experiences, both positive and negative. Through gentle movement and awareness, you can **release stored tension and emotional blocks**. This integration process allows you to move with greater ease, both physically and emotionally.

6. Individuality: Every body is unique, with its own history and needs. Somatic movement celebrates this **individuality**. There's no one-size-fits-all approach. You learn to listen to your body's unique signals and tailor your practice accordingly.

7. Non-Linear Journey: Don't expect instant results or linear progress. Somatic movement is a **non-linear journey**. There will be days of breakthroughs and days of frustration. The key is to be patient, kind to yourself, and celebrate small victories along the way.

8. Curiosity & Playfulness: Cultivate a sense of **curiosity and playfulness** in your practice. Experiment, explore, and have fun with movement. This playful attitude fosters engagement and makes learning more enjoyable.

9. Connection & Community: While somatic movement is often a personal journey, it can also be a powerful tool for **connection and community**. Sharing experiences and learning from others can deepen your understanding and enhance your practice.

10. Lifelong Practice: Somatic movement is not a quick fix, but a **lifelong practice**. As you continue to explore, you'll discover new layers of yourself and your movement potential. Embrace this journey of continuous learning and growth.

Remember, these are just guiding principles, not rigid rules. The beauty of somatic movement lies in its flexibility and adaptability. By incorporating these principles into your practice, you can embark on a transformative journey of self-discovery, cultivating a deeper connection between your mind and body, and unlocking a newfound sense of ease and well-being.

Unveiling the Science: Somatic Exercises Backed by Evidence

For centuries, somatic practices have been praised for their transformative benefits, promoting stress reduction, pain management, and improved well-being. But beyond anecdotal evidence, **can science substantiate these claims?** Absolutely! Recent research paints a compelling picture, revealing the potent impact of somatic exercises on various aspects of our physical and mental health.

1. Stress Reduction: Somatic exercises can effectively counteract the detrimental effects of stress on our bodies and minds. Studies show that practices like mindfulness meditation and gentle movement activate the **parasympathetic nervous system**, responsible for relaxation and recovery. This activation counterbalances the "fight-or-flight" response of the sympathetic nervous system, leading to lowered stress hormones, reduced anxiety, and improved sleep quality.

2. Pain Management: Chronic pain can be debilitating, both physically and emotionally. Somatic practices offer a promising approach to managing pain, often working alongside traditional therapies. Research suggests that these exercises can:

- **Increase self-awareness** of pain sensations, allowing individuals to manage them more effectively.
- **Reduce muscle tension** and improve flexibility, contributing to pain relief.
- **Promote the release of endorphins**, the body's natural pain relievers.

3. Trauma Recovery: The impact of trauma often lingers long after the emotional wounds have healed. Somatic exercises provide a safe and gentle way to address these stored tensions. Studies indicate that these practices can:

- **Facilitate the release of trauma-related tension** held in the body, easing physical and emotional discomfort.

- **Improve emotional regulation** by helping individuals connect with their bodies and process emotions in a safe space.
- **Empower individuals to reclaim a sense of agency** over their bodies and lives.

4. Enhanced Flexibility & Mobility: Somatic exercises differ from traditional stretching regimes by emphasizing gentle exploration and awareness. This approach proves beneficial for improving flexibility and mobility in several ways:

- **Increased awareness of movement limitations** allows for targeted and mindful stretches, avoiding overexertion and injury.
- **Gentle mobilization techniques** stimulate the nervous system and release tension, improving joint range of motion.
- **Enhanced body awareness** leads to more efficient and fluid movement patterns, reducing the risk of stiffness and pain.

5. Deeper Self-Awareness & Connection: Somatic exercises are not just about physical movement; they foster a deeper connection with the self. By focusing on internal sensations and emotions, you gain insights into your thoughts, patterns, and needs. This enhanced self-awareness empowers you to:

- **Make conscious choices** regarding your physical and emotional well-being.
- **Manage stress more effectively** by recognizing your body's early warning signs.
- **Develop greater self-compassion** by cultivating a kinder and more understanding relationship with yourself.

The Science Continues to Evolve:

While the research landscape for somatic exercises is vast and promising, it's constantly evolving. New studies are continually emerging, solidifying the scientific foundation of these practices and uncovering new benefits for various health conditions.

Remember, the science is just one lens through which to view the power of somatic exercises. Your own personal experience is equally important. By incorporating these practices into your life and observing their impact on your well-being, you can join the growing community discovering the transformative potential of moving with awareness and intention.

Unveiling the Diverse Landscape of Somatic Practices: A Journey Through Movement and Mind

The world of somatic practices is like a vibrant tapestry, woven with threads of movement, mindfulness, and self-discovery. Each thread, representing a unique type of practice, offers a different path towards a deeper connection with your body and mind. Let's explore some of the most prominent threads in this tapestry:

1. Feldenkrais Method: This gentle and introspective practice emphasizes small, mindful movements that explore your range of motion and habitual patterns. Through this exploration, you gradually learn to move with greater ease and efficiency, releasing tension and improving flexibility.

2. Alexander Technique: This method focuses on improving posture and movement habits by learning to release unnecessary muscle tension. Through verbal cues and gentle touch, practitioners learn to identify and release tension, leading to improved alignment, reduced pain, and greater awareness of their bodies.

3. Laban Movement Analysis: This method explores the language of movement, focusing on the dynamics, spatial relationships, and qualities of movement. By analyzing and experiencing these qualities, individuals gain a deeper understanding of their own movement patterns and how they can express themselves more authentically.

4. Body-Mind Centering (BMC): This practice explores the interconnectedness of the body's various systems and organs through movement and imagery. By focusing on specific anatomical structures and their relationships, you learn to move with more awareness and integrate your mind and body more deeply.

5. Rosen Method: This gentle and supportive practice focuses on releasing physical and emotional tension held in the body. Through mindful touch and verbal guidance, practitioners create a safe space for individuals to explore their emotions and release stored tension, leading to greater emotional well-being and physical ease.

6. Craniosacral Therapy: This gentle hands-on therapy focuses on the subtle rhythms and movements of the craniosacral system, believed to influence the central nervous system. By listening to these subtle movements, practitioners aim to support the body's natural healing processes and promote overall well-being.

7. Yoga: While not exclusively somatic, many yoga styles incorporate elements of mindfulness, breathwork, and gentle movement, making them valuable tools for somatic exploration. Practices like Hatha, Vinyasa, and Yin yoga offer various levels of intensity and focus, allowing you to find a style that resonates with your needs.

8. Pilates: This method emphasizes core strength, alignment, and controlled movements. While not traditionally considered somatic, some Pilates variations incorporate mindfulness and breathwork, creating a more holistic experience that can benefit both body and mind.

9. Dance Movement Therapy (DMT): This therapy uses dance and movement as tools for emotional expression, self-discovery, and healing. DMT can help individuals process trauma, improve communication skills, and cultivate a deeper connection to their bodies.

10. Mindfulness Meditation: While not technically a movement practice, incorporating mindfulness meditation into your somatic exploration can greatly enhance your awareness and deepen your connection to your body's subtle sensations. This practice allows you to observe your thoughts and emotions without judgment, creating a space for greater self-understanding and acceptance.

Remember: This list is not exhaustive, and new somatic practices are continually emerging. The key is to explore and find what resonates with you. Listen to your body, connect with your breath, and embark on a journey of movement and self-discovery with an open mind and a curious spirit.

Additional Tips:

- Consider your individual needs and preferences when choosing a practice.
- Seek qualified practitioners who are experienced in the specific method you choose.
- Start slowly and gently, allowing your body to adapt to the new movement patterns.
- Be patient and kind to yourself. The benefits of somatic practices unfold gradually over time.
- Embrace the journey of exploration and self-discovery, and witness the transformative power of moving with awareness and intention.

By embarking on this exploration of the diverse landscape of somatic practices, you unlock a doorway to a more mindful, connected, and empowered way of being. So, step onto the path, explore the different threads, and weave your own tapestry of movement, self-discovery, and well-being.

Chapter 4

Addressing Trauma Through Somatic Practices

The Echo of Trauma: Understanding its Impact on Body and Mind

Trauma, whether a single event or repeated experiences of emotional or physical distress, leaves its mark not just on our minds, but also on our bodies. It's like a ripple effect, disturbing the delicate balance between our physical and psychological well-being. To truly understand and heal from trauma, we must explore its multifaceted impact on both body and mind.

The Mind Under Siege:

The immediate impacts of trauma on the mind are evident:

- **Intrusive thoughts and memories:** Flashbacks, nightmares, and unwanted thoughts about the traumatic event can be relentless, causing anxiety and emotional distress.

- **Hypervigilance:** The nervous system remains on high alert, scanning for potential threats, leading to difficulty relaxing and feeling safe.
- **Emotional dysregulation:** Trauma can disrupt the ability to manage emotions, leading to irritability, anger outbursts, or emotional numbing.
- **Negative self-beliefs:** Shame, guilt, and a sense of worthlessness can develop, impacting self-esteem and relationships.

The Body Holds the Score:

Beyond the emotional realm, trauma manifests in various physical ways:

- **Chronic pain:** Muscle tension, headaches, and other pain syndromes can be rooted in unprocessed trauma held in the body.
- **Sleep disturbances:** Difficulty falling asleep, staying asleep, or nightmares can

be a common consequence of disrupted nervous system functioning.

- **Dissociation:** Feeling disconnected from one's body or emotions can be a coping mechanism developed during trauma.
- **Weakened immune system:** Chronic stress triggered by trauma can compromise the immune system, making individuals more susceptible to illness.
- **Gastrointestinal issues:** Digestive problems like irritable bowel syndrome can be linked to the stress response activated by trauma.

The Interconnected Dance:

It's crucial to understand that these impacts are not separate entities. The mind and body are intricately connected, and what affects one inevitably influences the other. For example, chronic pain can contribute to anxiety and sleep disturbances, further impacting emotional well-being. Similarly, negative self-beliefs can lead to avoidance behaviors that worsen physical symptoms.

Healing the Journey:

The good news is that healing from trauma is possible. By addressing both the mental and physical aspects of the experience, individuals can embark on a journey of recovery and reclaim their well-being. Here are some key approaches:

- **Trauma-informed therapy:** This specialized therapy helps individuals process and integrate their traumatic experiences in a safe and supportive environment.
- **Somatic practices:** Exercises like yoga, mindfulness meditation, and bodywork can help release stored tension in the body, improve emotional regulation, and cultivate self-awareness.
- **Physical activity:** Regular exercise releases endorphins, natural mood boosters, and promotes better sleep, aiding in stress management and emotional well-being.
- **Healthy lifestyle choices:** Prioritizing adequate sleep, nutritious food, and

relaxation techniques can support the body's natural healing processes.

- **Social support:** Connecting with supportive friends, family, or therapy groups can provide a sense of belonging and understanding.

Remember: Healing from trauma is a journey, not a destination. It requires patience, self-compassion, and the willingness to explore both the emotional and physical aspects of the experience. By understanding the interconnectedness of mind and body, individuals can break free from the limitations of trauma and reclaim their wholeness.

Somatic Exercises: Weaving the Threads of Healing after Trauma

Trauma leaves deep scars, not just on our minds, but also on our bodies. Flashbacks, intrusive thoughts, and emotional dysregulation are just the tip of the iceberg. Trapped tension, chronic pain, and a sense of disconnection from the body are equally significant yet often overlooked consequences. Somatic exercises, with their unique blend of mindfulness and gentle movement, offer a powerful tool to support the healing process after trauma. Here's how:

1. Releasing Stored Tension: Trauma triggers a fight-or-flight response, leading to muscle tension that gets locked in the body. Somatic exercises, through gentle movements and breathwork, help release this held tension. By focusing on body sensations and allowing them to soften, individuals can experience a physical and emotional release, easing pain and promoting relaxation.

2. Cultivating Embodied Awareness: Trauma can disconnect us from our bodies, making it difficult to identify and manage emotions. Somatic exercises foster embodied awareness, encouraging individuals to pay attention to subtle sensations, posture, and breath. This heightened awareness allows them to better understand their body's responses to emotions, facilitating emotional regulation and self-compassion.

3. Reclaiming Agency and Control: Trauma can leave individuals feeling helpless and out of control. Somatic exercises empower individuals to regain a sense of agency over their bodies. By learning to move with intention and awareness, they can make conscious choices about their physical experience, fostering a sense of empowerment and control that extends beyond the physical realm.

4. Building Resilience and Nervous System Regulation: Chronic hypervigilance and stress responses characteristic of trauma can be exhausting for the nervous system. Somatic exercises, with their emphasis on slow, gentle movements and mindful breathing, activate the parasympathetic nervous system, promoting relaxation and nervous system regulation. This helps individuals build resilience and better manage stress, promoting overall well-being.

5. Fostering Self-Compassion and Acceptance: Trauma can lead to harsh self-judgment and a critical inner voice. Somatic practices cultivate self-compassion by encouraging individuals to observe their bodies and sensations with curiosity and kindness. This non-judgmental approach fosters self-acceptance, a crucial foundation for healing and personal growth.

6. Creating a Safe Space for Processing: Somatic exercises are not just physical movements; they create a safe and supportive space for emotional exploration. By connecting with the body's sensations and movements, individuals can begin to process and release stored emotions, facilitating deeper healing and integration.

7. Promoting Connection and Community: Trauma can lead to isolation and disconnection. Somatic practices that involve group movement or even simply sharing experiences with others can foster a sense of connection and community. This sense of belonging and support can be invaluable for individuals navigating the healing journey.

Remember: Somatic exercises are not a magic bullet, but a powerful tool to support the healing process. They work best when combined with other forms of therapy and self-care practices. Additionally, it's crucial to find a qualified practitioner who understands trauma and can create a safe and supportive environment for exploration.

With patience, self-compassion, and a willingness to explore, somatic exercises can offer a path towards healing, integration, and reclaiming a sense of wholeness after trauma.

Specific Somatic Exercises for Trauma Recovery: A Path Towards Healing

While the benefits of somatic practices for trauma recovery are well-established, it's important to remember that individual experiences and needs vary greatly. Consulting a qualified therapist trained in trauma and somatic modalities is crucial to craft a personalized practice for your specific journey. However, here are some commonly used and adaptable exercises you can explore, adapted from various somatic approaches:

1. Body Scans:

- Lie down comfortably or sit with good posture. Close your eyes and bring your attention to your breath. Slowly scan your body, starting with your toes and moving upwards, noticing any sensations without judgment. Pay attention to areas of tension, tightness, or discomfort. Observe these sensations without trying to change them. Repeat the scan a few times, focusing on different areas each time.

2. Gentle Breathwork:

- Sit or lie down comfortably. Place one hand on your chest and the other on your belly. Focus on your breath, feeling the rise and fall of your belly with each inhale and exhale. Breathe slowly and deeply, aiming for longer exhalations. Notice any areas where your breath feels shallow or restricted. Allow your breath to be natural and effortless. Practice for a few minutes, gradually increasing the duration over time.

3. Progressive Muscle Relaxation:

- Tense and relax different muscle groups in your body, starting with your toes and working your way up. For example, clench your toes tightly for a few seconds, then release, noticing the difference in sensation. Repeat with different muscle groups, focusing on the contrast between tension and relaxation. Pay attention to how your body feels after releasing tension.

4. Grounding Exercises:

- Stand with your feet hip-width apart and imagine roots growing down from your feet into the earth. Feel the solidity and support of the ground beneath you. wiggle your toes and feel your connection to the ground. You can also try standing barefoot on grass or soil, feeling the texture and temperature beneath your feet.

5. Gentle Movement Exploration:

- Move your body slowly and mindfully, exploring different ranges of motion. Notice how your body feels with each movement. Focus on small and gentle movements, avoiding any that cause pain or discomfort. Pay attention to your breath and how it connects to your movement.

6. Creative Expression:

- Engage in activities like drawing, painting, or dance that allow you to express yourself nonverbally. Focus on the process of creating, rather than the final product. This can be a safe space to explore and release emotions related to your trauma.

Additional Tips:

- Start slowly and listen to your body. Don't push yourself beyond what feels comfortable.
- Focus on curiosity and exploration, rather than judgment or achieving specific outcomes.
- Practice regularly, even if it's just for a few minutes each day.
- Combine somatic exercises with other forms of trauma-informed therapy and self-care practices.
- Seek guidance from a qualified therapist trained in trauma and somatic modalities.

Remember, healing from trauma is a journey, not a destination. Be patient with yourself, celebrate small victories, and trust the process. Somatic exercises can be a powerful tool on your path towards reclaiming your well-being and living a life free from the limitations of trauma.

Chapter 5

Embarking on Your Somatic Journey: Addressing Common Concerns

Somatic exercises offer a unique and transformative approach to connecting mind and body, promoting well-being and healing. Yet, starting any new practice can come with uncertainties and anxieties. Let's address some common concerns you might have about embarking on your somatic journey:

1. "I'm not flexible or coordinated enough."

Somatic exercises are not about achieving impressive feats of flexibility or acrobatics. They focus on gentle, mindful movement and exploration, accessible to all regardless of fitness level or physical limitations. The emphasis is on awareness and sensation, not performance.

2. "I don't have time for another exercise routine."

Somatic practices are not about adding more pressure to your already busy schedule. Even starting with short, 5-minute sessions can make a significant difference. You can find exercises that fit seamlessly into your daily life, like mindful breathing while waiting for the kettle to boil or gentle stretches before bed.

3. "I'm worried about hurting myself."

Somatic practices prioritize safety and listening to your body. Certified practitioners can guide you through safe and appropriate movements based on your individual needs and limitations. Always start slowly and pay attention to any signals of discomfort. If anything feels uncomfortable, stop and adjust the movement or seek guidance from your practitioner.

4. "I'm not sure I can be comfortable with my own body."

Somatic practices cultivate self-compassion and acceptance. The focus is on observing your body with curiosity and non-judgment, not criticizing or trying to "fix" anything. This gentle exploration can foster a more positive and accepting relationship with yourself.

5. "I'm intimidated by the unfamiliar."

It's natural to feel unsure when trying something new. Start by exploring different types of somatic practices, like yoga, Pilates, or Feldenkrais, to find what resonates with you. Consider attending workshops or group classes to experience the practice in a supportive environment.

6. "I'm skeptical about the benefits."

While individual experiences vary, research supports the positive impact of somatic practices on stress reduction, pain management, trauma recovery, and overall well-being. Be open to exploring and see how it affects you personally. Remember, the benefits often unfold gradually, so be patient and trust the process.

7. "I think therapy would be more helpful."

Somatic practices can be a valuable complement to therapy, but they are not a replacement. If you're struggling with significant trauma or mental health challenges, seeking professional therapeutic guidance is crucial. However, somatic exercises can enhance the benefits of therapy by fostering deeper body awareness and promoting self-regulation.

8. "I don't know where to start."

Many resources are available to help you begin your somatic journey. Consider:

- Consulting a qualified practitioner trained in somatic modalities for personalized guidance.
- Participating in online workshops or classes offered by various organizations.
- Exploring online resources and educational videos on different types of somatic practices.
- Starting with simple exercises like mindful breathing or body scans at home.

Remember: Starting small, being patient, and listening to your body are key. Embrace the exploration, celebrate your progress, and allow yourself to experience the transformative power of connecting mind and body through somatic practices.

Additional Tips:

- Find a supportive community, whether online or in-person, to share your experiences and learn from others.
- Be patient and kind to yourself. Progress takes time, and there will be ups and downs.
- Celebrate small victories and acknowledge your commitment to taking care of yourself.
- Don't be afraid to ask questions and seek guidance when needed.

With an open mind and a willingness to explore, somatic practices can be a powerful tool for unlocking your full potential for well-being and a deeper connection to yourself.

Cultivating Sanctuary: Creating a Safe and Supportive Somatic Practice Environment

The journey of somatic exploration requires a foundation of safety and support, allowing you to delve into your body and emotions with trust and openness. Here are some key steps to cultivate a safe and supportive practice environment, whether you're working with a practitioner or embarking on a solo journey:

1. Choose Your Space Wisely:

- **Physical Comfort:** Select a quiet, clutter-free space where you won't be interrupted. Ensure comfortable temperature, adequate lighting, and ventilation.
- **Emotional Comfort:** Create an environment that feels calming and safe. Use soothing colors, scents, or music that resonates with you.

- **Eliminate Distractions:** Silence your phone, turn off notifications, and inform others to respect your practice time.

2. Cultivate Self-Compassion:

- **Non-Judgment:** Approach your practice with curiosity and kindness, not criticism. Observe your body sensations and emotions without judgment.
- **Acceptance:** Acknowledge your limitations and challenges with self-compassion. Celebrate small victories and progress, not just "perfect" outcomes.
- **Respecting Limits:** Listen to your body's signals. Stop any movement that causes pain or discomfort and adjust as needed.

3. Establish Safe Boundaries:

- **Clear Communication:** If working with a practitioner, voice any concerns or preferences before starting. Discuss your boundaries regarding touch, privacy, and the intensity of exercises.

- **Empowerment:** Remember, you have the right to stop any exercise or end the session if you feel uncomfortable or unsafe.
- **Support System:** Build a network of supportive friends, family, or a therapist who can provide emotional support and understanding during your journey.

4. Foster Mindful Presence:

- **Focus on Your Body:** Pay attention to your breath, sensations, and emotions without getting caught up in thoughts or worries.
- **Grounding Techniques:** Use practices like mindful breathing, visualization, or focusing on physical sensations in the present moment to anchor yourself in the here and now.
- **Gratitude:** Cultivate a sense of gratitude for your body and its abilities. This fosters a positive and appreciative relationship with yourself.

5. Create a Ritualistic Setting:

- **Setting Intentions:** Before starting your practice, set an intention for your session, whether it's relaxation, exploration, or releasing tension.
- **Warm-Up and Cool-Down:** Incorporate gentle stretches or movement sequences to prepare your body and mind for practice and ease yourself back into daily activities afterwards.
- **Post-Practice Reflection:** Take some time to reflect on your experience. Journaling your thoughts, feelings, and physical sensations can offer insights and deepen your understanding.

Additional Tips:

- **Connect with Nature:** Spending time outdoors can be grounding and calming, enhancing your somatic practice.
- **Explore Different Modalities:** Experiment with various types of somatic practices like yoga, meditation, or

bodywork to find what resonates most with you.

- **Seek Guidance:** Consider working with a qualified somatic practitioner, especially if you have specific needs or concerns.
- **Remember, Progress Takes Time:** Be patient with yourself. The benefits of somatic practices unfold gradually, so enjoy the journey of exploration and self-discovery.

By creating a safe and supportive environment, you empower yourself to embark on a transformative journey of somatic exploration, fostering deeper self-awareness, healing, and a profound connection with your mind and body.

Cultivating Sanctuary Within: The Power of Self-Compassion and Trust in Your Body

Our bodies are intricate vessels, carrying within them not just physical form, but also a wealth of emotions, experiences, and memories. Yet, navigating the complexities of human existence can often lead us to disconnect from our physical selves, fostering self-criticism and distrust. This is where the twin pillars of self-compassion and trust in your body emerge, offering a path towards healing, well-being, and a deeper connection with who we truly are.

The Radiance of Self-Compassion:

Imagine a close friend struggling with pain or self-doubt. What would your response be? Chances are, you'd offer kind words, understanding, and support. Extending this same compassion to ourselves is the essence of self-compassion. It's about acknowledging our challenges and imperfections with kindness and acceptance, rather than harsh judgment.

Why is self-compassion so crucial for our relationship with our bodies?

- **Breaking the Cycle of Self-Criticism:** Constant negativity towards our bodies can lead to shame, avoidance, and even self-harm. Self-compassion replaces this negativity with understanding, allowing us to listen to our bodies' needs and respond with care.

- **Embracing Vulnerability:** We all experience pain, discomfort, and limitations. Self-compassion allows us to acknowledge these vulnerabilities without judgment, fostering resilience and courage to face challenges.

- **Unlocking Forgiveness:** Holding onto past mistakes or negative experiences can create tension in our bodies. Self-compassion encourages forgiveness, releasing this tension and promoting emotional and physical well-being.

- **Building a Positive Relationship with Our Bodies:** When we treat ourselves with kindness and understanding, we cultivate a positive and respectful relationship with our bodies. This fosters appreciation for all that our bodies do for us, leading to better self-care and a stronger connection.

Building Trust in Your Body: A Path to Wholeness:

Our bodies are constantly communicating with us through sensations, emotions, and intuitive nudges. Yet, ignoring these signals can create a disconnect, leading to confusion and mistrust. Building trust in your body is about learning to listen to its messages and responding with respect.

How can we cultivate trust in our bodies?

- **Mindful Awareness:** Pay attention to your physical sensations, emotions, and intuitions throughout the day. Practice mindfulness exercises like meditation or body scans to become more attuned to your body's subtle messages.

- **Respecting Physical Limits:** Pushing our bodies beyond their limits can create discomfort and injury. Trusting your body means honoring its limitations and listening to its signals of fatigue or pain.
- **Responding to Needs:** When your body tells you it needs rest, nourishment, or movement, respond with care. Taking care of your physical needs builds trust and strengthens your body-mind connection.
- **Celebrating Strengths:** Acknowledge your body's unique abilities and strengths, whether it's your resilience, flexibility, or sensory perception. This fosters appreciation and a positive relationship with your physical form.
- **Letting Go of Comparisons:** Constantly comparing your body to others can fuel self-doubt and disconnect. Trusting your body means accepting it as it is, with its unique strengths, limitations, and beauty.

The Journey of Self-Compassion and Trust:

Developing self-compassion and trust in your body is a lifelong journey. There will be times when negativity creeps in, and moments when you doubt your body's messages. Be patient with yourself, remember that progress is not linear, and celebrate even small victories. With consistent practice and gentle self-care, you can cultivate a deeper connection with your body, fostering healing, well-being, and a sense of wholeness.

Additional Tips:

- Explore somatic practices like yoga, meditation, or bodywork to enhance body awareness and cultivate self-compassion.
- Surround yourself with supportive people who encourage self-acceptance and respect for your body.
- Seek professional help if you struggle with body image issues or negative self-talk.

- Remember, you are worthy of love and respect, just as you are.

By nurturing self-compassion and building trust in your body, you unlock a doorway to a more fulfilling and empowered life, where you move through the world with confidence, acceptance, and a deep appreciation for the incredible vessel that carries you.

Chapter 6

Creating a Safe Space: Preparing for Somatic Exercises:

Choosing the right environment and clothing

Choosing the right environment and clothing for your somatic exercises depends on several factors, including the specific type of exercise you're doing, your personal preferences, and any physical limitations you may have. Here's a breakdown to help you make informed choices:

Environment:

- **Temperature:** Aim for a comfortable temperature that won't distract you. Avoid being too hot or too cold, as this can affect your focus and comfort.
- **Lighting:** Choose natural light whenever possible, or create a soft, calming ambience with artificial lighting. Avoid harsh fluorescent lights.
- **Noise:** Find a quiet space free from distractions like loud music or

conversation. Some practices may incorporate calming sounds like nature recordings, but choose what works best for you.

- **Comfort and Safety:** Ensure the space is clean, well-ventilated, and free of obstacles. Choose a comfortable surface for lying down or sitting, like a yoga mat, blanket, or cushion.

Clothing:

- **Comfort and Movement:** Opt for loose-fitting, comfortable clothing that allows for freedom of movement without restriction. Avoid tight-fitting clothing that can pinch or chafe.
- **Natural Fabrics:** Choose breathable, natural fabrics like cotton or wool over synthetic materials that can trap heat and moisture.
- **Layering:** Consider layering your clothes so you can adjust to changing temperatures during your practice.

- **Footwear:** Some practices may require bare feet or socks, while others might allow comfortable shoes with good flexibility. Choose what feels best for you and the specific exercise.

Additional Tips:

- **Consider the time of day:** If you're practicing in the morning, opt for slightly warmer clothes, while evening practices might be more comfortable in lighter clothing.
- **Prioritize personal needs:** If you have any physical limitations or sensitivities, adapt the environment and clothing accordingly. For example, if you have cold feet, wear warm socks or bring a blanket.
- **Experiment and adjust:** Don't be afraid to experiment with different environments and clothing options to find what works best for you. Remember, the goal is to create a space that feels safe, comfortable, and conducive to your practice.

Here are some specific examples for different types of somatic practices:

- **Yoga:** You might prefer a room with warm temperatures, natural light, and calming music. Wear loose-fitting yoga pants or shorts and a comfortable top.
- **Meditation:** A quiet, dimly lit room is ideal. Wear comfortable clothing that won't distract you, like loose pants and a soft top.
- **Feldenkrais:** Choose a warm room with comfortable mats or blankets. Wear loose-fitting clothing that allows for easy movement.

Ultimately, the most important thing is to choose an environment and clothing that allows you to relax, focus, and fully engage in your somatic practice.

Setting Realistic Expectations and Intentions for Somatic Exercises: A Guide to Inner Exploration

Somatic exercises offer a powerful path towards self-discovery and well-being. However, setting unrealistic expectations and intentions can lead to frustration and disappointment. Here's how to cultivate realistic and empowering approaches for your journey:

Understanding Realistic Expectations:

- **Somatic practices are not magic bullets:** They require dedication, patience, and consistent practice. While some may experience immediate shifts, others might see subtle changes over time.
- **Progress is not linear:** There will be ups and downs, days where you feel great and others where you struggle. Celebrate small victories and remember, progress is not always visible.
- **Discomfort is part of the process:** Exploring bodily sensations can

sometimes bring up discomfort or buried emotions. Acknowledge these feelings with compassion and allow yourself to process them gently.

- **Comparison is the thief of joy:** Focusing on others' experiences can create unrealistic expectations for yourself. Remember, your journey is unique, and celebrating your own progress is key.

Crafting Empowering Intentions:

- **Focus on process, not outcome:** Instead of aiming for specific results, set intentions about the experience itself. For example, your intention could be to explore your body with curiosity or to practice self-compassion.
- **Start small and specific:** Instead of a broad goal like "become more flexible," set smaller, achievable intentions like "spend 5 minutes each day exploring my breath."
- **Be present and open:** Approach each practice with an open mind and curiosity.

Allow yourself to be surprised by what arises without clinging to expectations.

- **Honor your body's needs:** Listen to your body's signals and adjust your intentions accordingly. If you're feeling tired, rest instead of pushing yourself.

Additional Tips:

- **Start with a beginner-friendly practice:** Ease into somatic exercises with gentle options like mindful breathing or body scans.
- **Find a supportive community:** Connect with others who are practicing somatic exercises. Share experiences and encourage each other's journeys.
- **Track your progress:** Journaling or keeping simple notes can help you track your progress and celebrate small victories.
- **Seek guidance:** Consider working with a qualified somatic practitioner who can personalize your practice and support your journey.

Remember, the most important aspect is to approach your somatic exploration with kindness and patience. Embrace the process, celebrate small victories, and trust that you are on a path towards greater self-awareness and well-being. By setting realistic expectations and crafting empowering intentions, you can unlock the transformative potential of somatic practices and create a more fulfilling relationship with your body and mind.

Warming up before engaging in somatic exercises is crucial for preparing your body and mind for safe and effective exploration. While the specific warm-up routine may vary slightly depending on the specific somatic practice you choose (e.g., yoga, Feldenkrais), here are some general guidelines:

Gentle Movement & Activation:

- **Start with gentle movements to gradually increase your heart rate and blood flow.** Begin with small circles of your head, neck, wrists, and ankles. Include shoulder rolls, arm circles, and gentle stretches for your torso and legs.
- **Focus on mindful movement, paying attention to your breath and body sensations.** Avoid forceful movements or pushing yourself beyond your comfort zone.

Breathwork & Mindfulness:

- **Incorporate mindful breathing exercises like diaphragmatic breathing or alternate nostril breathing.** This helps calm the nervous system and promotes focus.
- **Take a few moments for quiet reflection or meditation.** This helps you connect with your body and intentions before starting the practice.

Specific Considerations:

- **If you have any physical limitations or injuries, consult a healthcare professional or qualified practitioner before starting any new exercise program.** They can advise you on suitable warm-up exercises and modifications.
- **Consider the environment and time of day.** If practicing outdoors in cold weather, spend a little more time warming up. If practicing in the evening, a gentler warm-up might be appropriate.

Here are some examples of warm-up exercises for different somatic practices:

- **Yoga:** Sun salutations, gentle twists, and lunges can be incorporated into your warm-up.
- **Meditation:** Start with mindful breathing exercises and gentle seated stretches.
- **Feldenkrais:** Begin with small, exploratory movements focusing on different body parts and their range of motion.

Additional Tips:

- **Don't forget to warm up your feet and ankles, especially if you'll be standing or moving around.** Ankle circles and toe wiggles can help.
- **Listen to your body and adjust the intensity of your warm-up accordingly.** Don't force anything that feels uncomfortable.
- **Remember, the warm-up is just the beginning.** Allow yourself to gradually

transition into your chosen somatic practice and maintain a mindful approach throughout.

By taking the time to warm up properly, you'll prepare your body and mind for a safe and enjoyable somatic exploration, maximizing your experience and minimizing the risk of injury.

Chapter 7

Exercises for Stress and Anxiety Reduction

Gentle Body Scans for Relaxation and Awareness: Embarking on Your Inner Journey

Body scans offer a powerful tool for cultivating relaxation, self-awareness, and deeper connection with your body. Here are three gentle body scans you can explore, each with varying lengths and focuses:

1. 5-Minute Mini-Scan for Busy Moments:

- **Find a comfortable position:** Lie down or sit with good posture, eyes closed or open.
- **Start with your breath:** Tune into your breath, noticing its rhythm and depth. Breathe slowly and naturally, without forcing anything.
- **Begin your scan:** Bring your awareness to your toes, feeling any sensations

without judgment. Gently scan upwards, noticing any areas of tension, relaxation, or discomfort. Observe, don't judge.

- **Scan your body in sections:** Move your awareness up your feet, legs, pelvis, lower back, abdomen, chest, arms, hands, neck, and head. Pay attention to temperature, pressure, and any subtle movements.
- **Bring your awareness back to your breath:** Take a few deep breaths, integrating the sensations from your scan.
- **Slowly open your eyes if closed and gently move your body.**

2. 10-Minute Deep Dive Scan for Relaxation:

- Follow the same steps as the 5-minute scan, starting with breath and comfortable positioning.
- **Spend more time on each body section:** As you scan, imagine sending a wave of relaxation through each area. Visualize tension melting away as you breathe deeply.

- **Pay attention to emotions:** Notice any emotions that arise during your scan. Acknowledge them without judgment and allow them to move through you with your breath.
- **Focus on gratitude:** As you finish your scan, express gratitude to your body for its strength and resilience.

3. 15-Minute Guided Scan for Emotional Exploration:

- Follow the same steps as the 10-minute scan, focusing on both physical and emotional sensations.
- **Ask yourself questions:** As you scan each body part, ask yourself questions like: "What emotions are present here?" "Is there any tension or discomfort?" "What does this area need?"
- **Offer compassion:** Send love and compassion to any areas holding pain or tension. Visualize them softening and releasing.

- **Journal your experience:** After your scan, spend a few minutes journaling about your experience. Note down any emotions, insights, or physical sensations that came up.

Additional Tips:

- **Use guided recordings:** Many free guided body scan recordings are available online or in meditation apps. Find one that resonates with you.
- **Customize your scan:** Feel free to adjust the length, focus, and wording of the scan to suit your needs and preferences.
- **Practice regularly:** The more you practice body scans, the deeper your awareness and relaxation will become.
- **Be patient:** Allow yourself time to explore and connect with your body through this gentle practice.

Remember, body scans are not about achieving a specific outcome or feeling. They are an invitation to explore your body and emotions with curiosity and kindness. By engaging in this practice regularly, you can cultivate a deeper sense of peace, self-compassion, and attunement to the wisdom of your inner world.

Deep Dives into Breathwork: Calming the Nervous System with Every Inhale

The breath, a seemingly simple act, holds immense power over our physical and mental well-being. When stress or anxiety grip us, our breathing becomes shallow and erratic, sending our nervous system into overdrive. Breathwork exercises offer a powerful antidote, utilizing specific breathing patterns to calm the nervous system and restore a sense of peace. Let's explore some potent techniques to navigate your journey:

1. Diaphragmatic Breathing (Belly Breathing):

- **The Master of Calm:** This fundamental technique engages your diaphragm, the primary muscle for breathing, promoting deep, slow breaths that activate the parasympathetic nervous system (PNS), the "rest and digest" response.
- **How to Practice:** Lie down or sit comfortably, placing one hand on your

belly and the other on your chest. As you inhale, feel your belly expand, not your chest. Exhale slowly, allowing your belly to gently deflate. Aim for 6-8 breaths per minute.

- **Benefits:** Reduces stress, anxiety, and blood pressure. Promotes relaxation, sleep, and improved digestion.

2. Box Breathing (Square Breathing):

- **Finding Stability:** This calming technique uses equal inhale, hold, exhale, and hold durations, creating a sense of structure and stability.
- **How to Practice:** Inhale for a count of 4, hold for 4, exhale for 4, and hold again for 4. Repeat for several minutes, adjusting the count as comfortable.
- **Benefits:** Promotes focus, mental clarity, and emotional regulation. Can help manage anxiety and panic attacks.

3. Alternate Nostril Breathing (Nadi Shodhana):

- **Balancing the Energy Flow:** This ancient practice balances the left and right hemispheres of the brain, promoting emotional and physical harmony.
- **How to Practice:** Close your right nostril with your thumb. Inhale through your left nostril, then close it with your ring finger. Exhale through your right nostril, open your left nostril, and inhale again. Repeat, alternating nostrils.
- **Benefits:** Reduces stress, anxiety, and headaches. Promotes emotional balance and mental clarity.

4. Guided Breathwork:

- **Navigating with Expertise:** Guided breathwork sessions can offer deeper exploration and support, especially for beginners.
- **How to Practice:** Seek out guided breathwork sessions led by qualified practitioners, either online or in person. These sessions often combine specific

breathing techniques with visualizations or affirmations.

- **Benefits:** Can provide deeper relaxation, emotional release, and insights. Offers support and guidance for personalized practice.

Additional Tips:

- **Practice regularly:** The benefits of breathwork grow with consistency. Aim for at least 5-10 minutes daily, or more if you find it helpful.
- **Find a comfortable environment:** Choose a quiet, distraction-free space where you can relax and focus on your breath.
- **Listen to your body:** Don't force any techniques that feel uncomfortable. Adjust the pace, duration, and intensity based on your needs.
- **Combine with other practices:** Breathwork can be integrated with mindfulness meditation, yoga, or other

relaxation techniques for a holistic approach.

Remember, breathwork is a journey, not a destination. Be patient, explore different techniques, and find what resonates with you. As you navigate the depths of your breath, you unlock a powerful tool for calming your nervous system, enhancing well-being, and accessing a deeper sense of inner peace.

Releasing Tension and Finding Ground: A Movement Sequence Journey

Tension, like a shadow, can cling to our bodies, causing discomfort and disconnection. Movement sequences offer a powerful tool to release this tension and promote grounding, connecting us to our physical selves and the present moment. Here, we explore two sequences: one for releasing tension and the other for promoting grounding.

1. Release and Flow: A Sequence for Tension Release:

- **Gentle Neck Rolls:** Start by rolling your head gently in a circle, feeling any tightness in your neck and shoulders. Repeat 5-10 times in both directions.

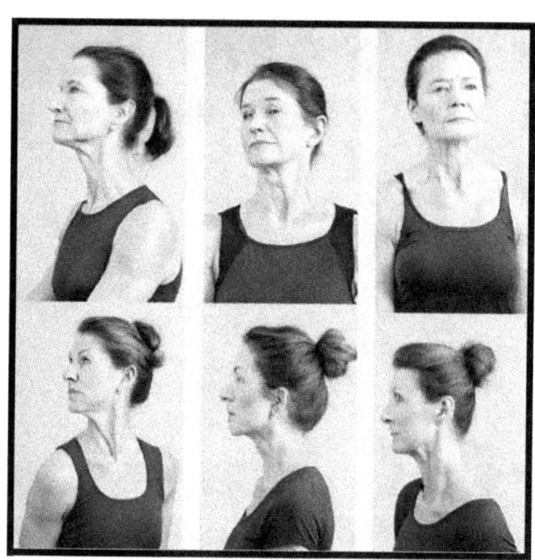

- **Arm Circles:** Extend your arms out to the sides and make small circles, forward first and then backward. Gradually increase the size of the circles, feeling the tension release in your shoulders and upper back. Repeat 5-10 times in each direction.

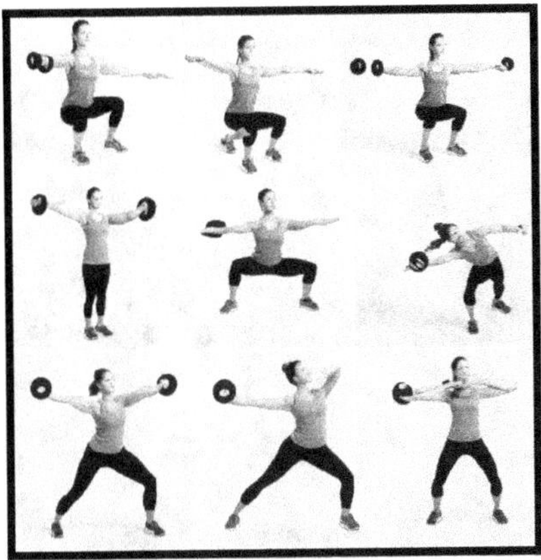

- **Pelvic Tilts:** Stand with your feet hip-width apart and gently tilt your pelvis forward and back, feeling the movement in your lower back and core. Repeat 5-10 times in each direction.

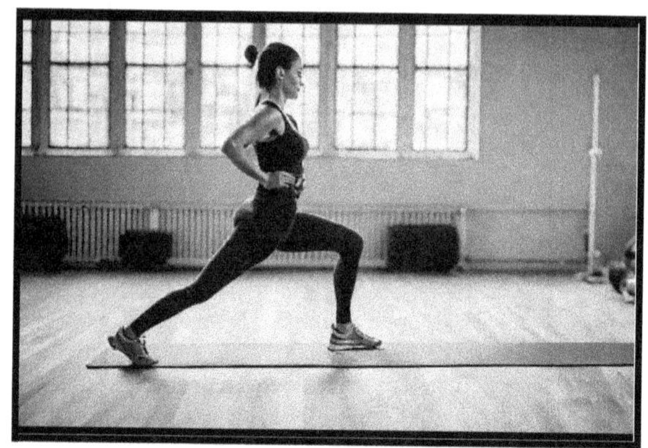

- **Spinal Twists:** Sit on the floor with your legs crossed or extended in front of you. Gently twist your upper body to the side, reaching your opposite hand to the floor behind you. Hold for a few breaths before switching sides. Repeat 3-5 times on each side.

- **Leg Swings:** Standing or sitting, gently swing one leg at a time, forward and backward, focusing on releasing tension in your hips and lower back. Repeat 5-10 times on each leg.

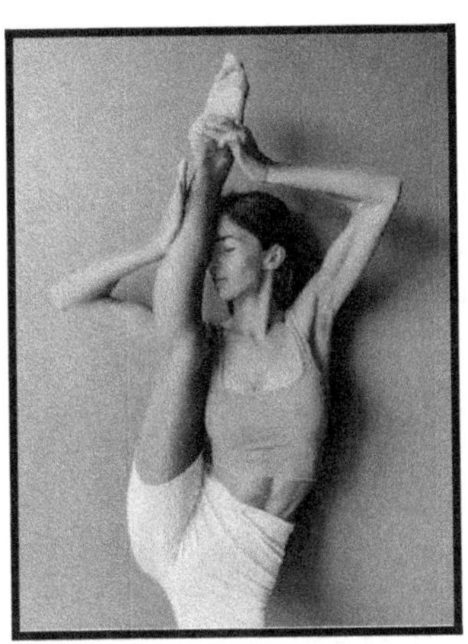

2. Finding Your Root: A Sequence for Grounding:

- **Tree Pose:** Start in Mountain Pose, then lift one foot off the ground and bring it to rest on your inner calf or ankle of the other leg. Focus on balancing and staying rooted. Hold for several breaths before switching sides.

- **Standing Meditation:** Stand tall, close your eyes, and focus on feeling your feet grounded into the earth. Imagine roots growing down from your feet and connecting you to the earth's core. Breathe deeply and stay for several minutes.

Remember:

- These are just examples, feel free to modify or create your own sequences based on your needs and preferences.
- Listen to your body and move gently, avoiding any pain or discomfort.
- Focus on your breath, connecting each movement to an inhale or exhale.
- Practice regularly for maximum benefits.
- Combine these sequences with other grounding practices like spending time in nature, mindful walking, or meditation.

By releasing tension and finding your ground through movement, you open yourself to a deeper sense of well-being, increased stability, and a calmer, centered presence in your daily life.

Chapter 8

Exercises for Trauma Recovery

Moving with Safety and Comfort: Trauma-Informed Practices for Somatic Exploration

For individuals who have experienced trauma, engaging in somatic practices can be a powerful tool for healing and self-discovery. However, it's crucial to approach these practices with sensitivity and understanding, prioritizing safety and comfort at every step. Here are some key principles and practices for creating a trauma-informed somatic experience:

1. Choice and Control:

- **Offer Choices:** Provide options for different types of movement, intensity levels, and environments. Allow individuals to choose what feels safe and comfortable for them.

- **Set Boundaries:** Clearly explain the boundaries of the practice and respect individual choices to participate or not.
- **Focus on Empowerment:** Encourage individuals to explore their bodies and sensations at their own pace. Avoid pushing or forcing any movement.

2. Predictability and Consistency:

- **Clear Explanations:** Provide clear and concise explanations of each movement or exercise before starting. Avoid ambiguity or surprises.
- **Routine and Ritual:** Establish a consistent routine and ritual for the practice, creating a sense of predictability and safety.
- **Grounding Techniques:** Offer grounding techniques like mindful breathing or visualization before, during, and after the practice to maintain a sense of stability.

3. Body Neutrality and Non-Judgment:

- **Non-Judgmental Language:** Avoid language that emphasizes "fixing" or "improving" the body. Use neutral terms and focus on exploring sensations without judgment.
- **Focus on Sensations, Not Appearance:** Encourage individuals to focus on internal sensations like breath, muscle tension, and emotional cues, rather than external appearances.
- **Respecting Personal Boundaries:** Respect individual boundaries regarding touch, proximity, and physical contact. Offer modifications if needed.

4. Trauma-Informed Modifications:

- **Offer Alternatives:** Provide alternative exercises or adaptations for individuals who may find certain movements triggering or uncomfortable.
- **Trigger Warnings:** If working with a group, consider offering trigger warnings before introducing specific exercises that might evoke trauma responses.

- **Trauma-Sensitive Environment:** Create a calm and quiet environment free from distractions or potential triggers.

Additional Tips:

- **Connect with a Trauma-Informed Practitioner:** Seek guidance from a practitioner trained in trauma-informed somatic practices who understands the unique needs of individuals who have experienced trauma.
- **Start Slowly:** Begin with short practice sessions and gradually increase the duration and intensity as comfort builds.
- **Focus on Breath:** Encourage a focus on mindful breath throughout the practice as a grounding and calming tool.
- **Celebrate Progress:** Acknowledge and celebrate any progress, no matter how small, as a step towards healing and self-compassion.
- **Remember, Healing is a Journey:** Healing from trauma takes time and

patience. Be kind to yourself and allow the process to unfold naturally.

By incorporating these principles and practices, you can create a safe and supportive environment for somatic exploration, fostering healing and empowerment for individuals who have experienced trauma. Remember, the most important aspect is to prioritize safety, respect, and individual needs, allowing each person to move through their own unique journey of self-discovery and well-being.

Embarking Within: Guided Visualizations for Emotional Release and Self-Compassion

Imagine a safe and nurturing space within you, where you can release emotional burdens and cultivate self-compassion. Guided visualizations offer a powerful tool to access this inner sanctuary, facilitating emotional release and fostering a deeper connection to your compassionate self. Here are two visualizations to explore:

1. Releasing Emotional Burdens:

- **Find a comfortable position:** Sit or lie down in a quiet space, ensuring you are comfortable and won't be disturbed.
- **Close your eyes and take a few deep breaths:** Focus on your breath, feeling the rise and fall of your chest or abdomen. Allow your body to relax with each inhale and exhale.
- **Imagine a safe space:** Visualize a place that feels safe and peaceful to you. It could be a real or imagined location, such

as a meadow, a beach, or a cozy library. Notice the details of this space: the colors, sounds, textures, and scents.

- **Encountering your burden:** Imagine a physical representation of your emotional burden, perhaps a heavy stone, a dark cloud, or a tangled knot. See it clearly in your mind's eye.

- **Releasing the burden:** Choose a way to release this burden. You might imagine carrying it to a safe place and leaving it there, dissolving it with light or warmth, or entrusting it to a trusted figure. Feel the relief and lightness as the burden disappears.

- **Filling your space with compassion:** Imagine a warm, golden light filling your safe space. This light represents self-compassion and acceptance. Allow it to wash over you, filling you with love and understanding.

- **Spend time basking in the light:** Stay in this space for as long as feels comfortable, soaking in the self-compassion. You can offer yourself kind words or affirmations.

- **Slowly return to your present moment:** When you're ready, gently bring your awareness back to your breath and your body. Open your eyes slowly, feeling refreshed and renewed.

2. Cultivating Self-Compassion:

- **Follow the same initial steps as above:** Find a comfortable position, close your eyes, and take a few deep breaths.

- **Imagine a younger version of yourself:** Bring to mind a younger version of yourself, perhaps a child or teenager. See them clearly in your mind's eye, noticing their emotions and needs.

- **Offer them compassion:** Imagine yourself as your current, compassionate self. Approach your younger self with kindness and understanding. Offer them words of comfort and love, just as you would to a dear friend.

- **Feel the compassion:** Notice how your younger self responds to your compassion. Allow yourself to feel the warmth and love radiating from you towards them.
- **Extend the compassion to yourself:** Now, imagine yourself receiving the same compassion from your future, wiser self. Feel the love and acceptance flowing towards you.
- **Become one with compassion:** Imagine yourself merging with the compassionate versions of yourself, past and future. Feel the wholeness and self-love radiating from within.
- **Carry the compassion forward:** Bring this sense of self-compassion with you as you open your eyes and return to your present moment. Allow it to guide your interactions with yourself and others.

Additional Tips:

- **Use guided visualization recordings:** Many free recordings are available online or in meditation apps. Find one that resonates with you and your current needs.

- **Personalize your visualizations:** Add details and imagery that feel meaningful to you. This will deepen your experience.
- **Practice regularly:** The more you practice guided visualizations, the easier it will become to access your inner sanctuary and cultivate self-compassion.
- **Remember, be patient:** Emotional release and self-compassion are journeys, not destinations. Be kind to yourself and trust the process.

By engaging in these visualizations, you can embark on a transformative journey of emotional release and self-compassion. Remember, the key is to create a safe and supportive space for yourself, approach your emotions with kindness, and allow your inner wisdom to guide you towards healing and well-being.

Somatic Meditations: Embodiment and Integration through Movement and Awareness

Somatic meditations offer a unique approach to processing and integrating experiences by engaging the body as an active participant in the healing process. By combining mindfulness with gentle movement and focused attention on physical sensations, these practices can unlock deeper understanding and facilitate emotional release. Here, we explore two powerful somatic meditations for processing and integration:

1. Body Scan for Integration:

- **Find a comfortable position:** Lie down or sit with good posture, eyes closed or open.
- **Begin with your breath:** Notice your natural breath, its rhythm and depth, without trying to control it. Feel your body rise and fall with each inhale and exhale.
- **Scan your body in stages:** Start with your toes, bringing your awareness to any sensations without judgment. Gently move your awareness upwards, noticing

any areas of tension, relaxation, or discomfort. Observe, don't judge.

- **Connecting sensations to experiences:** As you scan, consider if any memories, emotions, or thoughts arise related to specific body sensations. Don't force connections, simply observe what emerges.

- **Acknowledge and release:** If emotional responses arise, acknowledge them with compassion and allow them to flow through you without judgment. Imagine them releasing from your body with each exhale.

- **Integrate with gratitude:** As you finish your scan, express gratitude to your body for its wisdom and resilience. Carry the insights gained into your daily life.

2. Movement Exploration:

- **Find a spacious area where you can move freely:** Ensure you won't be disturbed and have comfortable clothing.

- **Start with gentle movements:** Begin with simple stretches, body rolls, or gentle walking. Focus on feeling your body move in space, without any specific goal or choreography.
- **Allow emotions to guide your movement:** As you move, let your emotions guide your expression. This could be through faster or slower movements, changes in direction, or more expressive gestures. Don't judge, simply allow yourself to move authentically.
- **Witnessing without judgment:** As you move, observe your emotions and sensations with a detached curiosity. Don't try to analyze or control them, simply be present with them.
- **Integration and closure:** After some time, gradually slow down your movements and come to a peaceful stillness. Reflect on your experience and integrate any insights gained into your understanding of the processed experience.

Additional Tips:

- **Use guided recordings:** Many guided somatic meditations are available online or in apps. Find one that resonates with your needs and preferences.
- **Modify for your needs:** Adapt the practices to your physical abilities and comfort level. Listen to your body and avoid pushing yourself.
- **Combine with other practices:** You can incorporate somatic meditations into your existing mindfulness or journaling practice for a more holistic approach.
- **Seek professional guidance:** If you're processing complex or traumatic experiences, consider working with a therapist trained in somatic therapy for additional support and guidance.

Remember, somatic meditations are a journey of self-discovery and exploration. Be patient, trust your body's wisdom, and allow yourself to experience the transformative power of integrating your experiences through mindful movement and awareness.

Chapter 9

Exercises for Enhancing Flexibility and Relieving Tension

Gentle Stretches and Mobilizations: Unlocking Your Body's Potential

Improving your range of motion (ROM) is beneficial for both physical and mental well-being. It can enhance your flexibility, reduce pain and stiffness, improve posture, and even boost your mood. However, forceful stretching or aggressive mobilizations can be counterproductive, leading to injury or discomfort. This guide focuses on gentle stretches and mobilizations, offering a safe and effective approach to increasing your ROM.

Key Principles:

- **Focus on quality over quantity:** Hold each stretch or mobilization for 20-30 seconds, focusing on deep, controlled movements. Avoid bouncing or pulling.

- **Listen to your body:** Stop if you feel any sharp pain, and ease off if you feel discomfort.
- **Breathe deeply:** Inhale as you prepare for the stretch, and exhale slowly as you deepen into it.
- **Be consistent:** Aim for 10-15 minutes of gentle stretches and mobilizations most days of the week.

Sample Stretches for Improved ROM:

Neck:

- **Gentle side bends:** Tilt your head towards each shoulder, feeling the stretch in your neck muscles.
- **Neck rolls:** Slowly roll your head in a circle, forward and backward.

Shoulders:

- **Arm circles:** Make small circles with your arms, forward and backward.

- **Shoulder shrugs:** Raise your shoulders towards your ears, hold for a few seconds, and then release.

Spine:

- **Cat-cow:** Arch your back as you inhale and round your back as you exhale, mimicking a cat and cow.
- **Spinal twists:** Sit or stand, twist your upper body to one side, and hold for a few breaths before switching sides.

Hips and Legs:

- **Leg swings:** Stand and gently swing one leg forward and backward, keeping your core engaged.
- **Knee circles:** Sit or lie down, circle your knees in both directions.
- **Butterfly stretches:** Sit with the soles of your feet together, gently press your knees down towards the floor.

Mobilizations:

- **Arm circles with self-massage:** Make small arm circles while gently massaging your shoulder muscles with your opposite hand.
- **Hip circles:** Stand with your hands on your hips, make small circles with your hips in both directions.
- **Ankle circles:** Sit or stand, circle your ankles in both directions.

Additional Tips:

- **Warm up before stretching:** Light cardio or dynamic stretches can prepare your muscles for deeper stretching.
- **Cool down after stretching:** Hold each stretch for a few breaths longer and perform gentle movements to prevent stiffness.
- **Target specific areas:** If you have specific tightness or limitations, focus your stretches and mobilizations on those areas.
- **Consult a healthcare professional:** If you have any injuries or medical

conditions, consult your doctor or therapist before starting a new stretching program.

By incorporating these gentle stretches and mobilizations into your routine, you can unlock your body's potential for improved range of motion, flexibility, and overall well-being. Remember, consistency and mindful practice are key to seeing and feeling the benefits.

Targeting Tension: Exercises for Specific Body Areas

Tension can build up in different areas of our bodies, causing discomfort, fatigue, and affecting our overall well-being. Luckily, specific exercises can help release tension and bring relief to targeted areas. Here's a guide to address common tension zones:

Neck & Shoulders:

- **Neck rolls:** Gently roll your head in a circle, forward and backward, for 10 repetitions each direction.
- **Shoulder shrugs:** Slowly raise your shoulders towards your ears, hold for 5 seconds, and release. Repeat 10 times.
- **Arm circles:** Make small circles with your arms, forward and backward, for 10 repetitions each direction.
- **Eagle arms:** Bring your arms in front of you, bend at the elbows, and clasp hands with opposite thumbs hooked. Wrap your forearms around each other, pressing

palms together. Hold for 30 seconds and repeat on the other side.

Back & Spine:

- **Cat-cow:** Start on hands and knees, arch your back as you inhale and round your back as you exhale. Repeat 10-15 times.
- **Spinal twists:** Sit or stand, twist your upper body to one side, reach your opposite hand behind you for support, and hold for 30 seconds. Repeat on the other side.
- **Child's pose:** Kneel on the floor, sit back on your heels, rest your forehead on the ground, and extend your arms forward. Hold for several minutes.

Hips & Legs:

- **Hip circles:** Stand with your hands on your hips, make small circles with your hips in both directions for 10 repetitions each.

- **Knee circles:** Sit or lie down, circle your knees in both directions for 10 repetitions each.
- **Figure-four stretch:** Lie on your back, cross one ankle over the opposite knee, and gently pull towards your chest. Hold for 30 seconds and switch sides.
- **Butterfly stretch:** Sit with the soles of your feet together, gently press your knees down towards the floor. Hold for 30 seconds.

Jaw & Face:

- **Jaw clenches:** Gently clench your jaw, hold for 5 seconds, and relax. Repeat 10 times.
- **Jaw stretches:** Open your mouth wide, hold for 5 seconds, and close. Repeat 10 times.
- **Facial massage:** Use your fingertips to gently massage your temples, forehead, and cheeks in circular motions.

Additional Tips:

- **Warm up before exercising:** Light cardio or dynamic stretches can prepare your muscles for deeper release.
- **Listen to your body:** Don't push through pain, stop if you feel uncomfortable and adjust the intensity.
- **Breathe deeply:** Focus on your breath throughout the exercises, inhaling as you prepare and exhaling as you release.
- **Repeat regularly:** Aim for 5-10 minutes of these exercises a few times a day for optimal results.
- **Consider professional help:** If chronic tension persists, consult a healthcare professional or physical therapist for personalized guidance.

Remember, releasing tension is an ongoing process. By incorporating these exercises and prioritizing relaxation techniques, you can create a more comfortable and stress-free life.

Soothing and Reviving: Self-Massage Techniques for Relaxation and Circulation

Self-massage offers a powerful tool for promoting relaxation, improving circulation, and boosting overall well-being. By applying gentle pressure and techniques to your muscles and tissues, you can release tension, stimulate blood flow, and induce a sense of calm. Here's an exploration of self-massage techniques for different areas:

Neck & Shoulders:

- **Thumb circles:** Use your thumbs to make small circles on your neck muscles, starting at the base and moving upwards. Repeat on both sides.
- **Finger kneading:** Knead your shoulder muscles with your fingertips, applying gentle pressure in circular motions.
- **Shoulder rolls:** Roll your shoulders forward and backward in slow, controlled movements.

Back & Spine:

- **Fist tapping:** Gently tap your fists on your back muscles, moving from top to bottom in a rhythmic motion.
- **Tennis ball massage:** Place a tennis ball between your back and a wall, lean against it, and use your body weight to apply pressure and roll up and down.
- **Foam rolling:** Use a foam roller to target larger muscle groups in your back, applying gentle pressure as you roll back and forth.

Legs & Feet:

- **Calf squeezes:** Squeeze your calves with your hands, moving upwards from your ankles towards your knees. Repeat on both legs.
- **Foot massage:** Apply pressure with your thumbs on the balls of your feet, working your way up your arches and toes.

- **Ankle circles:** Rotate your ankles in both directions, feeling the stretch in your calves and ankles.

General Tips:

- **Warm up with light movement:** Prepare your muscles with gentle stretches or light cardio before self-massage.
- **Use oil or lotion:** Apply lubricant to reduce friction and make the massage smoother.
- **Focus on your breath:** Breathe deeply and slowly throughout the massage, allowing your body to relax.
- **Listen to your body:** Don't push through pain, adjust pressure and techniques based on your comfort level.
- **Start gradually:** Begin with short sessions and gradually increase the duration as you become comfortable.
- **Target specific areas:** If you have tension in specific areas, focus your massage efforts on those spots.

- **Consider guided recordings:** Many online resources and apps offer guided self-massage routines for specific needs.

Additional Techniques:

- **Acupressure:** Apply gentle pressure to specific points on your body believed to stimulate energy flow and alleviate discomfort.
- **Gua Sha:** Use a smooth tool to gently scrape your skin, promoting circulation and releasing tension.
- **Self-myofascial release (SMR):** Use foam rollers, balls, or other tools to apply sustained pressure to trigger points and release muscle tension.

Remember, self-massage is a journey of self-discovery and personalized care. Experiment with different techniques, listen to your body's feedback, and find what brings you the most relaxation and relief. By incorporating self-massage into your routine, you can unlock a powerful tool for improving your physical and mental well-being.

Chapter 10

Alleviating Pain Through Somatic Exercises

Unveiling the Mystery: Understanding the Mind-Body Connection in Chronic Pain

Chronic pain, a persistent and often debilitating experience, is more than just a physical phenomenon. It's a complex interplay between the mind and body, where thoughts, emotions, and social factors intertwine to influence the experience of pain. Understanding this intricate mind-body connection is crucial for effective pain management.

The Symphony of Pain:

Imagine pain as a symphony with multiple instruments playing in harmony or discord. The physical injury or disease acts as the conductor, initiating the pain signal. But the intensity and perception of that pain are influenced by other "instruments":

- **Brain chemistry:** Neurotransmitters like serotonin and dopamine modulate pain perception. Stress and negative emotions can deplete these, amplifying pain signals.
- **Thoughts and beliefs:** Catastrophizing (fearing the worst) and negative self-talk can worsen pain, while positive self-affirmations and mindfulness can alleviate it.
- **Stress and anxiety:** Chronic stress activates the "fight-or-flight" response, tightening muscles and sensitizing the nervous system, leading to heightened pain.
- **Sleep:** Poor sleep disrupts pain regulation mechanisms and contributes to fatigue, further amplifying pain.
- **Social factors:** Lack of social support, isolation, and financial stress can exacerbate pain.

The Good News: Shifting the Melody:

The good news is that by understanding and addressing these mind-body connections, we can change the pain symphony. Here are some key strategies:

- **Mindfulness and meditation:** These practices cultivate present-moment awareness and acceptance, reducing emotional reactivity and improving pain management.
- **Cognitive-behavioral therapy (CBT):** CBT helps identify and modify negative thought patterns and behaviors that contribute to pain.
- **Relaxation techniques:** Deep breathing, progressive muscle relaxation, and guided imagery can reduce stress and muscle tension, easing pain.
- **Exercise:** Regular physical activity improves mood, sleep, and circulation, alleviating pain and promoting overall well-being.
- **Healthy sleep habits:** Prioritizing good sleep hygiene ensures your body has the resources to manage pain effectively.

- **Social support:** Building strong connections with loved ones provides emotional support and reduces stress, contributing to better pain management.

Remember:

- The mind-body connection is unique to each individual. What works for one person may not work for another.
- Finding the right combination of mind-body approaches is crucial for effective pain management.
- Be patient and persistent. Changing ingrained patterns takes time and effort.
- Seek professional help if you need guidance in navigating the mind-body connection and managing your chronic pain.

By recognizing the intricate relationship between your mind and body, you can unlock a wealth of powerful tools for managing chronic pain. Remember, you are not alone in this journey. With knowledge, support, and the right approach, you can find ways to lessen the impact of pain and reclaim a life filled with well-being.

Taming the Tiger: How Somatic Exercises Can Help Manage Pain

Chronic pain, a persistent and often debilitating companion, can significantly impact your life. While conventional treatments offer relief, exploring alternative approaches like somatic exercises can bring a whole new dimension to pain management. Let's delve into how these gentle yet powerful movements can help you tame the pain tiger and reclaim your well-being.

Understanding the Painful Equation:

Pain, like a complex equation, involves not just the physical injury but also a web of interconnected factors. These include muscle tension, stress, emotional responses, and even your perception of pain. Somatic exercises address these factors by:

- **Releasing Physical Tension:** Gentle movements and stretches target tight muscles and fascia, reducing pain-triggering tension and improving flexibility.

- **Calming the Nervous System:** By promoting relaxation and mindfulness, somatic exercises activate the parasympathetic nervous system, counteracting the stress response that amplifies pain.

- **Improving Body Awareness:** Somatic practices encourage you to tune into your body's sensations, allowing you to identify and address areas contributing to pain before they escalate.

- **Shifting Pain Perception:** By focusing on breath and movement instead of pain, somatic exercises help you break the pain cycle and shift your perception, reducing its emotional impact.

Exploring the Somatic Toolbox:

The beauty of somatic exercises lies in their versatility and adaptability. Here are some popular options:

- **Gentle Body Scans:** Focus on your body's sensations without judgment, noticing areas of tension and discomfort. This awareness can guide you towards targeted movements for release.
- **Mindful Movement:** Engage in slow, controlled movements, focusing on the breath and how each movement feels in your body. This cultivates body-mind connection and promotes relaxation.
- **Feldenkrais Method:** This method uses gentle movements and explorations to retrain movement patterns, improving flexibility, coordination, and pain management.
- **Alexander Technique:** Focusing on posture and alignment, this technique helps identify and release unconscious tension patterns that contribute to pain.

Beyond the Movements:

Remember, somatic exercises are not just about stretching and moving. They offer a holistic approach to pain management, including:

- **Breathing Techniques:** Deep, rhythmic breathing activates the relaxation response, calming the nervous system and reducing pain.
- **Meditation:** Mindfulness practices help cultivate present-moment awareness, reducing stress and emotional reactivity to pain.
- **Visualization:** Imagine yourself moving with ease and freedom, reducing the fear and anxiety that can amplify pain.

Starting Your Somatic Journey:

- **Find a Qualified Practitioner:** Consider working with a therapist trained in somatic therapy for personalized guidance and tailored exercises.
- **Start Slowly:** Begin with short sessions, gradually increasing duration and intensity as your comfort level increases.
- **Listen to Your Body:** Pay attention to your sensations and adjust exercises as needed. Don't push through pain.

- **Combine with Other Approaches:** Somatic exercises can complement other pain management strategies like medication, physical therapy, and cognitive-behavioral therapy.

Remember:

- **Pain management is a journey, not a destination.** Be patient and consistent with your practice to see lasting benefits.
- **Somatic exercises are not a magic bullet.** While they can be powerful tools, they may not eliminate pain entirely.
- **Celebrate small victories.** Acknowledge and celebrate every step forward in your pain management journey.

By incorporating somatic exercises into your life, you can unlock a new approach to managing pain. By addressing the mind-body connection and cultivating self-awareness, you empower yourself to move beyond the limitations of pain and reclaim a life filled with greater ease and well-being.

Targeting the Source: Specific Somatic Exercises for Different Types of Pain

While the principles of somatic movement remain consistent across various pain conditions, specific exercises can be tailored to address the unique needs of different types of pain. Here's an exploration of targeted practices for common pain areas:

Neck & Shoulder Pain:

- **Gentle neck rolls:** Slowly roll your head in a circle, forward and backward, focusing on releasing tension in your neck muscles.
- **Shoulder shrugs:** Gently raise your shoulders towards your ears, hold for a few seconds, and release. Repeat with slow, controlled movements.
- **Arm circles:** Make small circles with your arms, forward and backward, focusing on smooth and controlled movements.

- **Eagle arms:** Stretch your arms forward, bend at the elbows, and clasp hands with opposite thumbs hooked. Wrap your forearms around each other, pressing palms together. Hold for 30 seconds and repeat on the other side.

Back Pain:

- **Cat-cow:** Start on hands and knees, arch your back as you inhale and round your back as you exhale, mimicking a cat and cow. Focus on smooth transitions and connecting with your breath.
- **Spinal twists:** Sit or stand, twist your upper body to one side, reach your opposite hand behind you for support, and hold for 30 seconds. Repeat on the other side, focusing on gentle rotation without straining.
- **Child's pose:** Kneel on the floor, sit back on your heels, rest your forehead on the ground, and extend your arms forward. Hold for several minutes, allowing your body to relax and surrender.

- **Lying hip rotations:** Lie on your back, bring one knee towards your chest, and gently rotate your lower leg in small circles, both inward and outward. Repeat with the other leg.

Hip & Leg Pain:

- **Hip circles:** Stand with your hands on your hips, make small circles with your hips in both directions, focusing on controlled movements and avoiding sharp pain.
- **Knee circles:** Sit or lie down, circle your knees in both directions, gradually increasing the range of motion as your comfort level allows.
- **Figure-four stretch:** Lie on your back, cross one ankle over the opposite knee, and gently pull towards your chest. Hold for 30 seconds and switch sides, focusing on releasing tension in your glutes and piriformis muscles.
- **Wall squats:** Stand with your back against a wall, slide down as if sitting in a

chair, and hold for as long as comfortable. Gradually increase the hold time as your strength improves.

Headaches & Migraines:

- **Jaw clenches:** Gently clench your jaw, hold for 5 seconds, and relax. Repeat 10 times, focusing on releasing tension in your jaw muscles.
- **Temple massage:** Use your fingertips to apply gentle pressure and circular massage to your temples, focusing on relieving pressure and promoting relaxation.
- **Cooling eye compress:** Place a cool, damp cloth over your eyes for 10-15 minutes, allowing the coolness to soothe and reduce tension headaches.
- **Neck stretches:** Perform gentle neck stretches like side bends and gentle rotations, focusing on releasing tension from the muscles that can contribute to headaches.

Additional Tips:

- **Always listen to your body:** Don't push through pain, adjust exercises based on your comfort level, and modify them if needed.
- **Warm up before exercising:** Light cardio or dynamic stretches can prepare your muscles for deeper movements.
- **Breathe deeply:** Focus on your breath throughout the exercises, inhaling as you prepare and exhaling as you release.
- **Consistency is key:** Aim for regular practice, even if it's just for a few minutes each day.
- **Consult a healthcare professional:** If you have any underlying medical conditions or experience sharp pain, consult your doctor or therapist before starting any new exercise program.

Remember, finding the right somatic exercises for your specific pain needs may require exploration and experimentation. Be patient, listen to your body, and enjoy the journey towards a more pain-free and well-being-filled life.

Chapter 11

Standing Tall with Ease: Understanding the Power of Good Posture for Stress and Pain Management

Our posture, often an afterthought, plays a crucial role in both our physical and mental well-being. Good posture not only prevents musculoskeletal pain but also contributes significantly to stress reduction and overall health. Let's delve into the intricate relationship between posture, stress, and pain, and explore how cultivating good posture can empower you to move through life with greater ease and resilience.

The Body-Mind Connection:

Our bodies and minds are intricately linked. Poor posture, characterized by slumped shoulders, rounded back, and forward head, can trigger a cascade of negative effects:

- **Muscular Tension:** Slouching tightens muscles, leading to discomfort, fatigue, and pain in the neck, shoulders, back, and even headaches.

- **Restricted Breathing:** Compressed chest and abdomen restrict your ability to breathe deeply, limiting oxygen intake and contributing to anxiety and stress.
- **Reduced Energy:** Poor posture disrupts blood flow and circulation, leaving you feeling sluggish and drained.
- **Negative Self-Perception:** Slumping can project low confidence and hinder your mood, while good posture can boost self-esteem and create a more positive outlook.

The Antidote: The Power of Good Posture:

Maintaining good posture, with a tall spine, relaxed shoulders, and balanced weight distribution, offers a wealth of benefits:

- **Reduced Pain and Tension:** Proper alignment relieves muscle strain, improves circulation, and reduces pain in the back, neck, and shoulders.

- **Enhanced Energy and Breathing:** Improved posture opens your chest and abdomen, allowing for deeper breaths, increased oxygen intake, and boosting energy levels.
- **Improved Mood and Confidence:** Good posture projects confidence and self-assurance, positively impacting your mood and overall well-being.
- **Lower Stress Response:** Proper alignment activates the parasympathetic nervous system, promoting relaxation and reducing the body's stress response.

Cultivating Good Posture:

Making small but consistent changes can significantly improve your posture. Here are some tips:

- **Mindfulness:** Pay attention to your posture throughout the day, especially when sitting or standing for extended periods.

- **Stretching and Strengthening:** Regular stretching and strengthening exercises can improve flexibility, core strength, and muscular balance, contributing to good posture.
- **Ergonomics:** Ensure your workspace promotes good posture with an adjustable chair, proper monitor height, and keyboard placement.
- **Movement Breaks:** Get up and move around frequently throughout the day to prevent stiffness and promote better alignment.
- **Seek Guidance:** Consider working with a physical therapist or posture expert for personalized assessment and targeted exercises.

Beyond the Physical:

Remember, good posture is not just about aesthetics; it's about empowering yourself to move through life with greater ease and resilience. The benefits extend beyond the physical, impacting your mental and emotional well-being as well. By incorporating these practices and cultivating awareness, you can unlock the transformative power of good posture and experience a life filled with less pain, more energy, and increased confidence.

Additional Tips:

- Start small and gradually integrate posture-conscious practices into your routine.
- Be patient, changing ingrained habits takes time and effort.
- Celebrate your progress, no matter how small, as you journey towards better posture.
- Remember, good posture is not about rigidity, it's about finding a comfortable, balanced alignment that feels good for your body.

By understanding the powerful link between posture, stress, and pain, you can embark on a journey towards a healthier, happier, and more empowered you. Stand tall, breathe deeply, and move with ease!

Strengthening Your Core & Aligning Your Body: A Guide to Powerful Exercises

A strong core is the foundation for a healthy body. It provides stability, supports good posture, and helps reduce pain and injury risk. Additionally, improving your alignment can enhance your core strength and ensure your body functions optimally. Here's a comprehensive guide to exercises that strengthen your core and improve your alignment:

Strengthening the Core:

1. Plank: This classic exercise engages your entire core, including your abs, glutes, and back muscles. Start in a push-up position with your forearms on the ground and your body in a straight line from head to heels. Hold for 30 seconds to 1 minute, depending on your fitness level. Gradually increase the hold time as you get stronger. **2. Bird Dog:** This exercise targets your core and strengthens your glutes and back muscles. Start on all fours with your hands under your shoulders and knees under your hips.

Extend one arm forward and the opposite leg straight back, keeping your core engaged and your back flat. Hold for a few seconds, then switch sides. Repeat 10-15 times per side. **3. Dead Bug:** This exercise is great for targeting deep core muscles. Lie on your back with your knees bent and feet flat on the floor. Keep your lower back pressed into the ground and slowly extend one arm and the opposite leg straight out, keeping your core engaged. Hold for a few seconds, then switch sides. Repeat 10-15 times per side. **4. Side Plank:** This variation of the plank targets your obliques and hips. Lie on your side with your elbow directly under your shoulder and your legs stacked or staggered. Lift your hips off the ground, forming a straight line from head to heels. Hold for 30 seconds to 1 minute per side.

Improving Alignment:

1. Cat-Cow: This yoga pose helps mobilize your spine and improve flexibility. Start on all fours with your hands under your shoulders and knees under your hips. As you inhale, arch your back and look up. As you exhale, round your back and tuck your chin to your chest. Repeat 10-15 times. **2. Spinal Twists:** This exercise helps release tension and improve spinal mobility. Sit or stand with your legs hip-width apart. Twist your upper body to one side, reaching your opposite hand behind you for support. Hold for 30 seconds, then switch sides. Repeat 5-10 times per side. **3. Wall Slides:** This exercise helps improve your posture and shoulder alignment. Stand with your back against a wall and your feet hip-width apart. Walk your hands up the wall as you slide your spine down, keeping your core engaged and your back flat against the wall. Slide back up and repeat 10-15 times. **4. Foam Rolling:** Self-myofascial release with a foam roller can help improve your posture and flexibility by releasing tight muscles and fascia. Use a foam roller to target your back, glutes, and hamstrings, applying gentle pressure and rolling for 30-60 seconds per area.

Additional Tips:

- **Focus on quality over quantity:** Perform each exercise with proper form, even if you can only do a few repetitions at first.
- **Warm up before exercising:** Light cardio or dynamic stretches can prepare your muscles for the workout.
- **Breathe deeply:** Inhale as you prepare for the exercise and exhale as you release.
- **Listen to your body:** Don't push through pain, modify exercises as needed, and stop if you experience discomfort.
- **Be consistent:** Aim for at least 2-3 core and alignment exercises most days of the week.
- **Consult a healthcare professional:** If you have any injuries or medical conditions, talk to your doctor or physical therapist before starting a new exercise program.

By incorporating these exercises and tips into your routine, you can strengthen your core, improve your alignment, and experience the benefits of a healthier, more balanced body.

Remember, consistency and proper form are key to success!

Cultivating Graceful Awareness: Techniques for Mindful Movement and Posture Awareness

Mindful movement and posture awareness are powerful tools for enhancing your physical and mental well-being. By integrating mindfulness into your everyday movements, you can cultivate a deeper connection with your body, improve your posture, and reduce stress and pain.

The Benefits of Mindful Movement:

- **Improved Posture:** By paying attention to your body's sensations, you can identify and adjust poor posture habits, leading to better alignment and reduced pain.
- **Reduced Stress and Anxiety:** Focusing on your breath and movements can quiet your mind, reducing anxiety and promoting relaxation.
- **Enhanced Body Awareness:** Mindful movement increases your awareness of

your physical sensations, allowing you to identify areas of tension and discomfort.

- **Greater Enjoyment of Movement:** By focusing on the present moment, you can find joy in simple movements and unlock a deeper appreciation for your body's capabilities.

Techniques for Mindful Movement:

- **Body Scans:** Lie down comfortably and focus on each part of your body, noticing any sensations without judgment. This practice helps you identify areas of tension and release.
- **Mindful Walking:** As you walk, pay attention to the sensations in your feet, legs, and body with each step. Notice your breath and the rhythm of your movement.
- **Focus on Breath:** During any activity, focus on your breath, feeling the rise and fall of your chest and abdomen. This anchors you in the present moment and promotes mindfulness.

- **Slow Down:** Instead of rushing through movements, slow down and pay attention to each step or action. This increases awareness and allows for adjustments.
- **Engage Your Senses:** When moving, pay attention to your surroundings – the sights, sounds, and smells. This enriches your experience and grounds you in the present moment.

Techniques for Posture Awareness:

- **Regular Check-ins:** Throughout the day, pause and check your posture. Are your shoulders relaxed? Is your spine aligned? Are you sitting or standing tall?
- **Posture Reminders:** Set reminders on your phone or use posture apps that alert you to adjust your posture.
- **Mirrors and Photos:** Place mirrors strategically to see your posture or take photos to track your progress.
- **Stretch and Release:** Regularly stretch tight muscles that contribute to poor

posture, such as your chest, neck, and shoulders.

- **Strengthening Exercises:** Exercises that target your core, back, and glutes can improve your posture and support your body better.

Additional Tips:

- **Start small:** Choose one or two techniques to focus on at first and gradually incorporate more as you get comfortable.
- **Be patient:** Changing ingrained habits takes time and practice.
- **Don't judge yourself:** Accept your current posture without judgment and focus on making gradual improvements.
- **Find a supportive community:** Join a mindful movement class or online group for encouragement and motivation.
- **Celebrate your progress:** Acknowledge and celebrate even small changes in your posture and awareness.

By integrating these techniques into your daily life, you can cultivate a deeper connection with your body, improve your posture, and experience the joy of mindful movement. Remember, mindfulness is a journey, not a destination. Enjoy the process and embrace the transformative power of mindful movement and posture awareness.

Chapter 11

Your 28-Day Somatic Plan

Week-by-Week Exercise Breakdown for Different Goals:

Goal: Improve Overall Fitness

Week 1:

- **Cardio:** 30 minutes of moderate-intensity cardio 3 times a week (e.g., brisk walking, swimming, cycling).
- **Strength Training:** 2 full-body strength training sessions (e.g., bodyweight exercises, light weights).
- **Flexibility:** 10-15 minutes of static stretching daily.

Week 2:

- Increase cardio duration to 35 minutes per session.
- Add 1-2 sets to each strength training exercise.

- Try dynamic stretches before your workouts and static stretches afterwards.

Week 3:

- Increase cardio duration to 40 minutes per session.
- Focus on compound exercises for strength training (e.g., squats, lunges, push-ups).
- Add 1-2 new exercises to your routine.

Week 4:

- Increase cardio intensity to a slightly higher level.
- Try split routines, targeting different muscle groups each day.
- Consider incorporating yoga or Pilates for flexibility and core strength.

Goal: Build Muscle Mass

Week 1:

- 3 strength training sessions focusing on major muscle groups (legs, chest, back, shoulders, arms) with 3 sets of 8-12 repetitions per exercise.

- 20-30 minutes of moderate-intensity cardio 2-3 times a week.
- Prioritize proper form and technique over heavier weights.

Week 2:

- Increase weight or resistance to maintain the same challenge.
- Add supersets or drop sets to your workouts for increased intensity.
- Focus on progressive overload by gradually increasing weight, reps, or sets.

Week 3:

- Try different rep ranges (e.g., 6-8 reps for heavier weight, 12-15 reps for lighter weight).
- Incorporate rest-pause sets or negatives for additional muscle stimulation.

- Ensure adequate protein intake (0.8-1 gram per pound of bodyweight) for muscle growth.

Week 4:

- Consider adding a fourth strength training session if progress stalls.
- Try advanced techniques like pre-exhaustion or post-exhaustion sets.
- Ensure proper rest and recovery between workouts (48-72 hours for major muscle groups).

Goal: Increase Flexibility

Week 1:

- 20-30 minutes of dynamic stretching before workouts and static stretches after.
- Focus on major muscle groups and tight areas (e.g., hamstrings, quads, shoulders).
- Hold each stretch for 30-60 seconds, breathing deeply.

Week 2:

- Try yoga or Pilates classes for a structured flexibility routine.
- Add self-massage with a foam roller or massage balls to release tension.
- Hold each stretch slightly longer, aiming for 60-90 seconds.

Week 3:

- Explore different yoga styles, focusing on flexibility-focused options like Yin yoga.
- Incorporate active stretches, where you move slowly through the range of motion.
- Consider consulting a physical therapist or yoga instructor for personalized guidance.

Week 4:

- Try partner stretches to assist with deeper stretches.
- Use props like straps or blocks to increase accessibility of stretches.
- Celebrate your progress by noticing increased ease of movement and range of motion.

Remember:

- Listen to your body and rest when needed.
- Warm up before and cool down after each workout.
- Stay hydrated throughout the day.
- Track your progress and adjust your routine as needed.
- Most importantly, have fun and enjoy the process!

This is just a starting point, and you can customize your workouts based on your individual needs and preferences. Always consult a healthcare professional before starting any new exercise program.

Integrating Somatic Practices: A Guide to Embodiment and Well-being

Somatic practices offer a unique approach to cultivating self-awareness, improving movement, and enhancing overall well-being. Here are some extensive tips for integrating them into your life:

1. Start Small and Gradually Integrate:

- Don't overwhelm yourself! Begin with short, focused practices for 10-15 minutes daily. Gradually increase duration and frequency as you become comfortable.
- Explore different somatic modalities like yoga, dance, Feldenkrais, or bodywork, and choose ones that resonate with you.

2. Cultivate Curiosity and Awareness:

- Approach each practice with a sense of curiosity and exploration. Focus on how your body feels, not on achieving "perfect" postures or movements.

- Pay attention to your breath, sensations in your muscles, and any areas of tension or discomfort.

3. Listen to Your Body and Modify:

- There's no one-size-fits-all approach. Adapt exercises to fit your abilities and limitations. Don't push through pain, and modify as needed.
- Use props like blocks, bolsters, or chairs to support your body and make movements accessible.

4. Breathe Deeply and Connect with Your Inner World:

- Somatic practices often emphasize conscious, deep breathing. Focus on your breath, feeling its rise and fall, and use it to anchor yourself in the present moment.
- Allow your breath to guide your movements, creating a sense of flow and connection between your body and mind.

5. Find a Supportive Community:

- Consider joining a somatic class or workshop to learn from experienced instructors and connect with others on this journey.
- Sharing your experiences and challenges with others can be motivating and enriching.

6. Integrate Somatic Awareness into Daily Life:

- Pay attention to your posture and movement throughout the day. Notice how you sit, stand, and walk, and make adjustments when needed.
- Take mindful breaks and use simple somatic exercises to manage stress and tension.
- Be playful! Explore movement with joy and curiosity, and enjoy the process of rediscovering your body.

Additional Tips:

- **Set realistic goals:** Focus on progress over perfection, and celebrate small victories.
- **Be patient:** Change takes time. Be kind to yourself and trust the process.
- **Don't be afraid to experiment:** Try different practices and find what works best for you.
- **Use technology:** Explore apps, online resources, and guided meditations to support your practice.
- **Most importantly, have fun!** Somatic practices should be enjoyable, not stressful.

Remember, integrating somatic practices into your life is a journey, not a destination. Embrace the process, connect with your body, and enjoy the many benefits it has to offer!

Conclusion

Embracing the Somatic Journey

As we conclude this exploration of the vast and transformative world of somatic practices, it's important to remember that it's not just about exercises or techniques. It's about embarking on a journey of **embodiment and self-discovery**. It's about cultivating a deeper awareness of your body, its sensations, and its connection to your mind and emotions.

By integrating these practices into your life, even in small, mindful ways, you can unlock a wealth of benefits:

- **Reduced stress and anxiety:** Through breathwork, gentle movements, and self-awareness, you can learn to release tension and cultivate inner peace.
- **Improved physical health:** Somatic practices can enhance flexibility, posture,

and overall body awareness, reducing pain and promoting physical well-being.

- **Increased self-confidence:** As you connect with your body and its capabilities, you build trust and respect for yourself, leading to greater self-confidence.
- **Enhanced creativity and problem-solving:** By attuning to your body's subtle cues, you can tap into a deeper level of intuition and creative thinking.
- **A richer connection to life:** By embodying your experience, you can cultivate a deeper appreciation for the present moment and your place in the world.

Remember, this journey is unique to you. There is no right or wrong way to practice. Start with curiosity, listen to your body, and be patient with yourself. The rewards of a conscious, connected life are worth the effort.

So, take a deep breath, step into your body, and begin your own somatic adventure. You might be surprised by the transformations that await you!

Bonus

https://screenpal.com/watch/cZnZDCVKIyy

Video link for tutorials